AF823811

Official Journal of

European Society for Paediatric Endocrinology

ESPE European Society for Paediatric Endocrinology

SLEP
Sociedade Latino-Americana de Endocrinologia Pediátrica

APPES
Asia Pacific Pediatric Endocrine Society

HORMONE RESEARCH

From Developmental Endocrinology to Clinical Research

Founded 1970 as 'Hormones' by M. Marois
Continued by J. Girard (1976–1995); M.B. Ranke (1996–2003)

KARGER

Printed in Switzerland on acid-free and non-aging paper (ISO 9706) by Reinhardt Druck, Basel

Appears monthly: 2 volumes per year (12 issues)

Guidelines for Authors

Aim and Scope

'Hormone Research' aims to provide rapid publication of clinical investigations, mini reviews and novel insights from clinical experience, as well as experimental and methodological work related to paediatric and adolescent endocrinology. Correspondence is welcome, but publication of letters is at the discretion of the editors.

Submission

Manuscripts written in English should be submitted using the online submission website at:

www.karger.com/hre

or sent as e-mail attachment (the preferred word-processing package is MS-Word) to the Editorial Office:

hre@karger.ch

Prof. P. Czernichow
S. Karger AG
Editorial Office 'Hormone Research'
P.O. Box
CH–4009 Basel (Switzerland)
Tel. +41 61 306 1437
Fax +41 61 306 1434

They should be accompanied by a signed copyright transfer statement (please see submission website). The names and addresses of four experts in the appropriate area of research should accompany each manuscript. Selected scientist(s) will be invited to act as referee(s).

Main Sections

1. *Original papers*
   Any original papers on hormone research are accepted; we particularly welcome papers on developmental and clinical research.
2. *Mini reviews*
   Most mini reviews are submitted upon invitation. However, the editors are open to unsolicited mini reviews. Authors planning such a mini review are requested to contact the Editorial Office with an outline of the intended mini review. All mini reviews are subject to peer review. The guidelines for the mini reviews can be found at **www.karger.com/hre_guidelines#11.**
3. *Novel insights from clinical practice*
   We invite contributions to this section that provide novel insight into a clinical problem. We recognise the value of case reports and thus submissions can be based around a case or a number of similar cases. The *most important* aspect of the presentation is that it should provide a new perspective on a recognised clinical scenario or may represent an entirely new clinical condition. The novel aspects of the case(s) may be in the phenotype, the presentation, the investigation and/or the management. This category replaces the previous case report section.
   We propose that a highlighted box containing one or two bullet points on **'Established facts'** and **'Novel insights'** be placed on the first page of the report. This reinforce the novelty of the clinical observation.
   The manuscript should be presented with an abstract (up to 200 words), brief introduction, case or case series description and results, followed by a discussion. No limits on length or number of references are imposed. Statements for the highlighted box should also be included.

Conditions

All manuscripts are subject to editorial review. The names and addresses of four experts in the appropriate area of research should accompany each manuscript. Selected scientist(s) will be invited to act as referee(s). Manuscripts are received with the explicit understanding that they are not under simultaneous consideration by any other publication. Submission of an article for publication implies the transfer of the copyright from the author to the publisher upon acceptance. Accepted papers become the permanent property of 'Hormone Research' and may not be reproduced by any means, in whole or in part, without the written consent of the publisher.
It is the author's responsibility to obtain permission to reproduce illustrations, tables, etc. from other publications.

Arrangement

Title page: The first page of each paper should indicate the title, the authors' names, the institute where the work was conducted, and a short title for use as running head.
NB: Authors wishing to preserve the phonetic meaning of diacritics (PubMed reduces diacritics to their root characters) must spell their names accordingly when submitting manuscripts (e.g. Müller should be Mueller).

Full address: The exact postal address of the corresponding author complete with postal code must be given at the bottom of the title page. Please also supply phone and fax numbers, as well as e-mail address.

Key words: For indexing purposes, a list of 5 key words in English is essential.

Abstract: Each paper needs an abstract of up to 200 words. It should be structured as follows:

Background/Aims:	What is the major problem that prompted the study?
Methods:	How was the study done?
Results:	Most important findings?
Conclusion:	Most important conclusion?

Footnotes: Avoid footnotes. When essential, they are numbered consecutively and typed at the foot of the appropriate page.

Tables and illustrations: Tables and illustrations (both numbered in Arabic numerals) should be prepared on separate pages. Tables require a heading and figures a legend, also prepared on a separate page. Due to technical reasons, figures with a screen background should not be submitted. When possible, group several illustrations on one block for reproduction (max. size 180 × 223 mm) or provide crop marks.

Color illustrations
Online edition: Color illustrations are reproduced free of charge. In the print version, the illustrations are reproduced in black and white. Please avoid referring to the colors in the text and figure legends.
Print edition: Up to 6 color illustrations per page can be integrated within the text at CHF 760.– per page.

References: In the text identify references by Arabic numerals [in square brackets]. Material submitted for publication but not yet accepted should be noted as 'unpublished data' and not be included in the reference list. The list of references should include only those publications which are cited in the text. Do not alphabetize; number references in the order in which they are first mentioned in the text. The surnames of the authors followed by initials should be given. There should be no punctuation other than a comma to separate the authors. Preferably, please cite all authors. Abbreviate journal names according to the Index Medicus system. (Also see International Committee of Medical Journal Editors: Uniform requirements for manuscripts submitted to biomedical journals. N Engl J Med 1997;336:309–315.)

Examples
(a) Papers published in periodicals: Sun J, Koto H, Chung KF: Interaction of ozone and allergen challenges on bronchial responsiveness and inflammation in sensitised guinea pigs. Int Arch Allergy Immunol 1997;112:191–195.
(b) Papers published only with DOI numbers: Theoharides TC, Boucher W, Spear K: Serum interleukin-6 reflects disease severity and osteoporosis in mastocytosis patients. Int Arch Allergy Immunol DOI: 10.1159/000063858.
(c) Monographs: Matthews DE, Farewell, VT: Using and Understanding Medical Statistics, ed 3, revised. Basel, Karger, 1996.
(d) Edited books: Parren PWHI, Burton DR: Antibodies against HIV-1 from phage display libraries: Mapping of an immune response and progress towards antiviral immunotherapy; in Capra JD (ed): Antibody Engineering. Chem Immunol. Basel, Karger, 1997, vol 65, pp 18–56.

Reference Management Software: Use of EndNote is recommended for easy management and formatting of citations and reference lists.

Digital Object Identifier (DOI)

S. Karger Publishers supports DOIs as unique identifiers for articles. A DOI number will be printed on the title page of each article. DOIs can be useful in the future for identifying and citing articles published online without volume or issue information. More information can be found at www.doi.org.

Page Charges

There is no page charge for papers of 4 or fewer printed pages (including tables, illustrations and references). Each additional complete or partial page is charged to the author at CHF 650.–. The allotted size of a paper is equal to approx. 12 manuscript pages (including tables, illustrations and references). As the page charges are waived in any case for the first paper each year to be published by a member of ESPE, authors who are members of the ESPE should so indicate on the title page.

Proofs

pdf proofs are sent to the corresponding author and should be returned with the least possible delay.

Reprints

Order form and price list is sent with the pdf proofs. Orders submitted after the issue is printed are subject to considerably higher prices.

KARGER

Fax +41 61 306 12 34
E-Mail karger@karger.ch
www.karger.com

The Guidelines for Authors are available at:
www.karger.com/hre_Guidelines

HORMONE
RESEARCH

General Information

ISSN Print Edition: 0301–0163
ISSN Online Edition: 1423–0046

Journal Homepage: www.karger.com/hre

Publication Data: 'Hormone Research' is published 12 times a year. Volumes 71 and 72, each with 6 issues, appear in 2009.

Disclaimer: The statements, opinions and data contained in this publication are solely those of the individual authors and contributors and not of the publisher and the editor(s). The appearance of advertisements in the journal is not a warranty, endorsement, or approval of the products or services advertised or of their effectiveness, quality or safety. The publisher and the editor(s) disclaim responsibility for any injury to persons or property resulting from any ideas, methods, instructions or products referred to in the content or advertisements.

Subscription Rates: Subscriptions run for a full calendar year. Prices are given per year.

Personal subscription:

Print or Online	Print+Online combined
CHF 1575.–	CHF 1665.–
EUR 1125.–	EUR 1189.–
USD 1500.00	USD 1586.00

postage and handling (added to print and print+online)
CHF 75.60 Europe, CHF 113.40 Overseas
EUR 54.–
USD 107.40

Institutional subscription:

Print or Online	Print+Online combined
CHF 3150.–	CHF 3466.–
EUR 2250.–	EUR 2476.–
USD 3000.00	USD 3300.00

postage and handling (added to print and print+online)
CHF 94.80 Europe, CHF 141.60 Overseas
EUR 67.20
USD 134.40

Airmail surcharge: CHF 96.– / USD 91.20

Discount subscription prices:
Lawson Wilkins Society; ISPAD;
Schweizerische Gesellschaft für Endokrinologie.
Subscription included in membership fee for members of the European Society for Paediatric Endocrinology (ESPE); Sociedade Latino-Americana de Endocrinologia Pediátrica (SLEP); Asia Pacific Pediatric Endocrine Society (APPES).

Back Volumes and Single Issues: Information on availability and prices of single print issues and print or electronic back volumes can be obtained from Customer Service at *service@karger.ch.*

Bibliographic Indices: This journal is regularly listed in bibliographic services, including *Current Contents®* and PubMed/MEDLINE.

Photocopying: This journal has been registered with the Copyright Clearance Center (CCC), as indicated by the code appearing on the first page of each article. For readers in the US, this code signals consent for copying of articles for personal or internal use, or for the personal or internal use of specific clients, provided that the stated fee is paid per copy directly to
Copyright Clearance Center Inc.
222 Rosewood Drive
Danvers, MA 01923 (USA)
A copy of the first page of the article must accompany payment. Consent does not extend to copying for general distribution, for promotion, for creating new works, or for resale. In these cases, specific written permission must be obtained from the copyright owner,
S. Karger AG, P.O. Box
CH–4009 Basel (Switzerland).

Subscription Orders:
Orders can be placed at agencies, bookstores, directly with the Publisher or further Karger offices or representatives:

S. Karger AG
Medical and Scientific Publishers
P.O. Box
CH–4009 Basel
Switzerland
(for courier services only:
Allschwilerstrasse 10
CH–4055 Basel)
Tel. +41 61 306 11 11
Fax +41 61 306 12 34
E-Mail karger@karger.ch
www.karger.com

France:
Librairie Medi-Sciences Sarl
36, bd de Latour-Maubourg
75007 Paris
France
Tél. +33 (0) 1 45 51 42 58
Fax +33 (0) 1 45 56 07 80
E-Mail librairie@medi-sciences.fr
www.medi-sciences.fr

Germany:
S. Karger GmbH
Postfach
79095 Freiburg
Deutschland
(Hausadresse: Lörracher Strasse 16A
79115 Freiburg)
Tel. +49 761 45 20 70
Fax +49 761 45 20 714
E-Post information@karger.de
www.karger.de

India, Bangladesh, Sri Lanka:
Panther Publishers Private Ltd.
33, First Main
Koramangala First Block
Bangalore 560 034
India
Tel. +91 80 25505 836
Tel. +91 80 25505 837
Fax +91 80 25505 981
E-Mail panther_publishers@vsnl.com
www.pantherpublishers.com

Japan:
Karger Japan, Inc.
Yushima S Bld. 3F
4-2-3, Yushima, Bunkyo-ku
Tokyo 113-0034
Japan
Tel. +81 3 3815 1800
Fax +81 3 3815 1802
E-Mail publisher@karger.jp

China, Taiwan and Malaysia:
Karger China
Suite 409, Apollo Building
1440 Central Yan An Road
Shanghai 200040
China
Tel. +86-21-6133 1861
Fax +86-21-6133 1862
E-Mail karger.ray@gmail.com

South America and Central America:
Cranbury International LLC
7 Clarendon Ave., Suite 2
Montpelier, VT 05602
USA
Tel. +1 802 223 6565
Fax +1 802 223 6824
E-Mail
eatkin@cranburyinternational.com
www.cranburyinternational.com

United Kingdom, Ireland:
S. Karger AG
c/o London Liaison Office
4 Rickett Street
London SW6 1RU
United Kingdom
Tel. +44 (0) 20 7386 0500
Fax +44 (0) 20 7610 3337
E-Mail uk@karger.ch

USA:
S. Karger Publishers, Inc.
26 West Avon Road
P.O. Box 529
Unionville, CT 06085
USA
Toll free: +1 800 828 5479
Tel. +1 860 675-7834
Fax +1 860 675-7302
E-Mail karger@snet.net

Change of Address:
Both old and new address should be sent to the subscription source.

KARGER

Fax +41 61 306 12 34
E-Mail karger@karger.ch
www.karger.com

The Journal Home Page is available at:
www.karger.com/hre

HORMONE
RESEARCH

Juvenile Idiopathic Arthritis: Clinical Picture, Mechanisms of Disease and Effects of Growth Hormone Treatment

Experts Conference, May 25–26, 2008, Chantilly, France

Guest Editors
Paul Czernichow, Paris
Günther Dannecker, Stuttgart

26 figures, 6 in color, and 7 tables, 2009

KARGER

Basel · Freiburg · Paris · London · New York · Bangalore · Bangkok · Shanghai · Singapore · Tokyo · Sydney

Disclaimer

Pfizer initiated and funded the Juvenile Idiopathic Arthritis Experts Conference; however, the organization of the program and content was developed by a Scientific Board (the Board).

The Board is comprised of specialists who provide scientific and planning oversight for the overall Program. Specifically, the Board develops the scientific program content. Its members are recognized authorities in the field of endocrinology and rheumatology.

The presenters received payment from Pfizer for their presentations, but Pfizer has not had any editorial control over the content. The content of the Conference reflects the scientific opinions of the individual presenters and may not necessarily reflect the opinion of Pfizer, or any of its subsidiaries, partners or employees.

Disclosure Statement Guest Editors

P.C. has acted as a consultant, independent contractor, and/or speaker/teacher for Pfizer and Ipsen for which he has received consulting fees and honoraria.

G.E.D. declares membership on advisory committees or review panels for Wyeth, Pfizer and Bristol-Meyers Squibb for which he has received honoraria.

S. Karger
Medical and Scientific Publishers
Basel • Freiburg • Paris • London •
New York • Bangalore • Bangkok •
Shanghai • Singapore • Tokyo • Sydney

Printed in Switzerland
on acid-free and non-aging paper (ISO 9706) by
Reinhardt Druck, Basel
ISBN 978–3–8055–9292–5

KARGER

Fax +41 61 306 12 34
E-Mail karger@karger.ch
www.karger.com

Vol. 72, Suppl. 1, 2009

HORMONE
RESEARCH

Contents

KARGER

Fax +41 61 306 12 34
E-Mail karger@karger.ch
www.karger.com

Access to full text and tables of contents, including tentative ones for forthcoming issues:
www.karger.com/hre_issues

Introduction

HORMONE
RESEARCH

Horm Res 2009;72(suppl 1):1–3
DOI: 10.1159/000229756

Published online: November 27, 2009

Growth and Development Abnormalities in Children with Juvenile Idiopathic Arthritis: Treatment and Prevention

Paul Czernichow

Department of Endocrinology and Growth Diseases, Hôpital Necker-Enfants Malades, Paris, France

In 1897, in the Transactions of the Royal Medical and Surgical Society of London, Sir George Frederic Still described for the first time the devastating consequences on growth and development of a special form of childhood arthritis: 'A remarkable feature in these cases is the general arrest of development that occurs when the disease begins before the second dentition. A child of twelve and a half years would easily have been mistaken for six or seven years while another of four years looked more like two and a half or three years.' Half a century later, the introduction of glucocorticoid therapy radically improved the course of Still's disease (now called juvenile idiopathic arthritis [JIA]) and alleviated the pain so frequently experienced by affected children. However, glucocorticoids were soon found to worsen the slowing of growth and development. A Cushing-like appearance became a clinical feature of severe long-lasting JIA. Nevertheless, the deleterious effects of JIA on growth were recognized long before the advent of glucocorticoid therapy. Clearly, the growth arrest often seen in patients with severe JIA is not only due to glucocorticoid therapy, but also to disease-related factors. Nearly 100 years after the seminal description by Still, a possible link between severe inflammation and growth arrest was suggested: overproduction of an inflammatory cytokine was found to adversely affect the growth plate, leading or contributing to the growth impairment.

Improved understanding of the pathogenetic mechanisms of JIA has led to new treatments, most notably, biologic agents. Whether glucocorticoids still have a place in this new treatment era remains debatable; a definitive answer will probably await the accumulation of additional experience with the newer drugs. To date, selected patients with severe inflammation still require glucocorticoid therapy in combination with biologic agents.

Paediatric endocrinologists have long sought to overcome the problem of growth impairment in patients with chronic diseases. Growth is delayed in many diseases such as chronic renal failure, cystic fibrosis, and diabetes. Close collaboration between the specialist in charge of the underlying disease and the paediatric endocrinologist has led to substantial progress. In May 2008, a group of paediatric rheumatologists and endocrinologists met to discuss the impact of JIA on growth and the means of treating or preventing the developmental abnormalities so frequently observed in this disease. Numerous field specialists shared their experiences. The proceedings

KARGER

Fax +41 61 306 12 34
E-Mail karger@karger.ch
www.karger.com

0301–0163/09/0727–0001$26.00/0

Accessible online at:
www.karger.com/hre

Prof. Paul Czernichow
Pediatric Department
Hôpital des Enfants Malades
149 rue de Sèvres, FR–75743 Paris Cedex 15 (France)
Tel. +33 674 293 814, Fax +33 140 031 987, E-Mail paul.czernichow@nck.aphp.fr

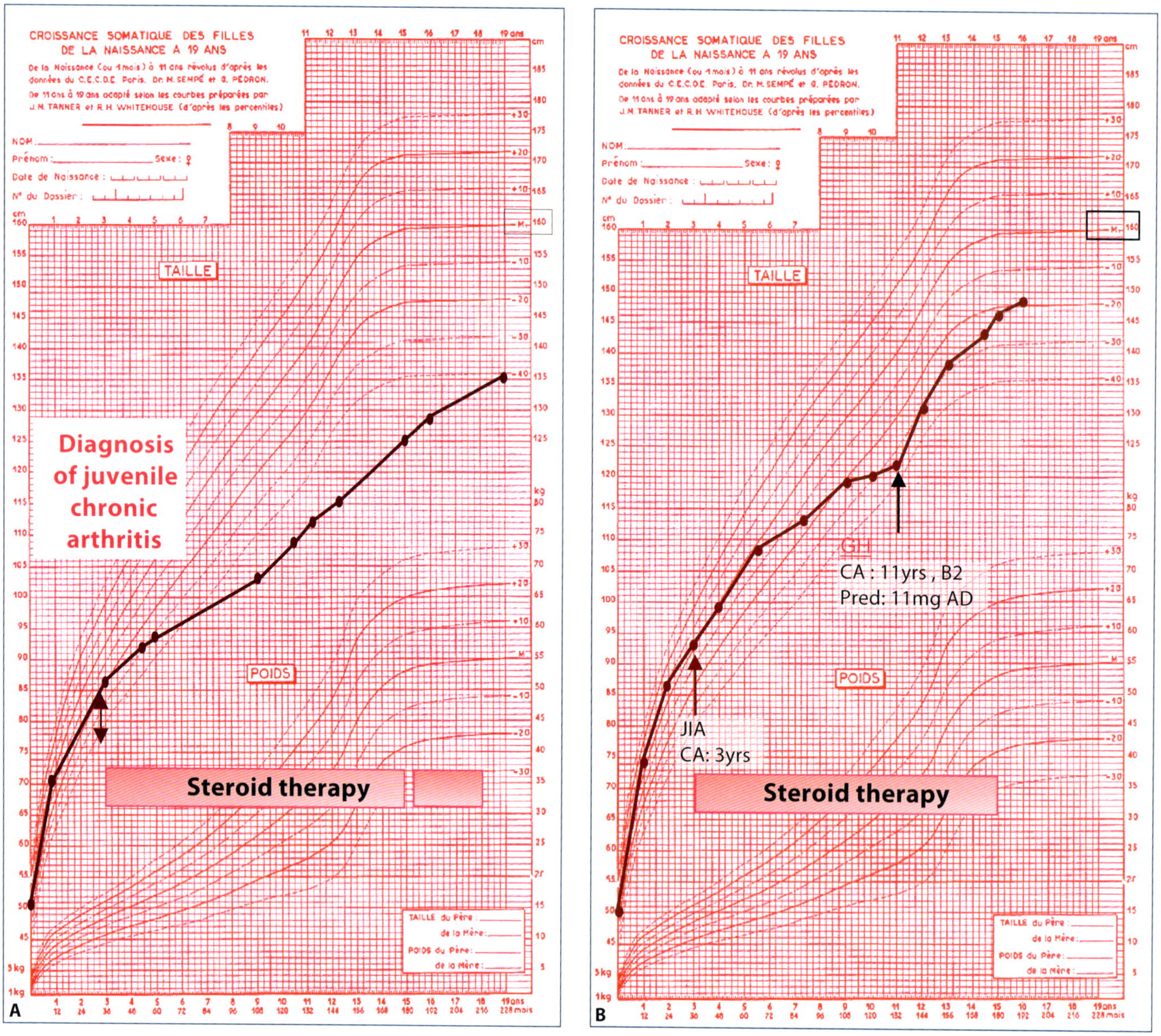

Fig. 1. Comparison on final height in three patients with JIA receiving different courses of treatment. All three patients were diagnosed with JIA of similar severity and were receiving similar dosage of corticosteroids. Growth curve **A** describes the growth of a patient treated 20 years ago with the devastating effect of the disease (and of the treatment) on the adult height of this patient (4 SD below target height). The two other curves describe the growth in patients receiving GH therapy. Growth curve **B** is from a patient who was treated with GH several years after disease onset and shows that GH therapy stops the deleterious effect of the disease on the growth velocity by allowing some catch-up growth (adult height still below target height). By contrast, growth curve **C** shows that when treated with GH shortly after disease onset, growth velocity is nearly normal allowing the patient to achieve a near-normal adult height.

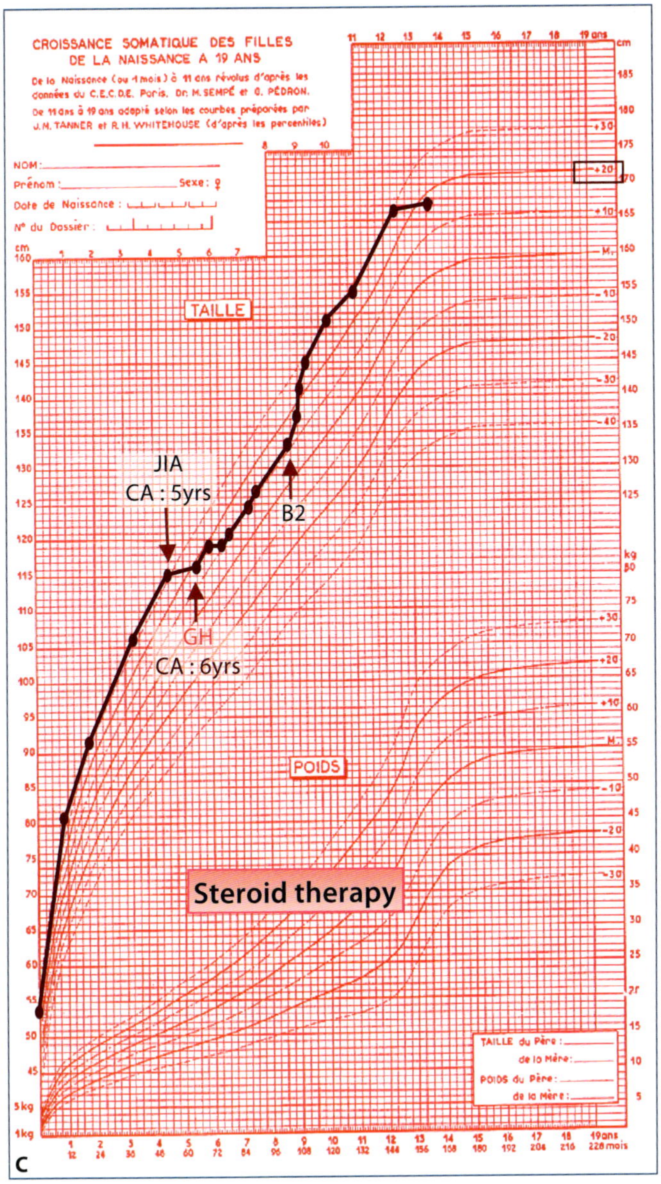

from this meeting constitute the first comprehensive overview of growth and developmental abnormalities in patients with JIA. They provide a clear picture of the situation from the points of view of both the rheumatologist and the endocrinologist.

The possibility that growth hormone (GH) may deserve a place in the therapeutic armamentarium for JIA was first considered several decades ago. In 1979, a German group led by Otfried Butenandt reported the effects of open-label GH therapy in 20 patients with JIA; several other studies were published subsequently. However, only within the last decade have randomized controlled trials established that GH therapy improves not only growth, but also body composition in children with JIA. Figure 1 compares the growth curves of three different patients: the first, from a patient given continuous glucocorticoid therapy 30 years ago for severe JIA; the second, from a patient in whom GH was administered several years after evolution of the disease and corticosteroid administration, and the third, from a patient with similar disease severity receiving glucocorticoid therapy who was treated with GH shortly after disease onset. The comparison shows that GH therapy prevents the deleterious effects of high-dose glucocorticoid therapy on growth.

Clearly, much has been gained from the active research conducted during the intervening 30 years. We are grateful to the specialists who have contributed to this important field of paediatrics. We hope the readers will find these proceedings helpful for understanding, treating, and preventing the developmental abnormalities seen in children with inflammatory joint disease. We are also extremely grateful to Pfizer for sponsoring the meeting in Paris and the publication of the proceedings.

HORMONE RESEARCH

Horm Res 2009;72(suppl 1):4–12
DOI: 10.1159/000229757

Published online: November 27, 2009

Juvenile Idiopathic Arthritis: Classification, Clinical Presentation and Current Treatments

Günther E. Dannecker[a] Pierre Quartier[b]

[a]Department of Pediatric Rheumatology, Olgahospital, Klinikum Stuttgart, Stuttgart, Germany; [b]Université Paris-Descartes and Unité d'Immuno-Hématologie et Rhumatologie Pédiatriques, Hôpital Necker-Enfants Malades, Paris, France

Key Words
Juvenile idiopathic arthritis · Classification · Presentation · Treatment

Abstract

Background: The term juvenile idiopathic arthritis (JIA) describes a clinically heterogeneous group of arthritides. The onset in all subgroups is before 16 years of age, but each group presents with different clinical signs and symptoms. The cause of the disease is unknown, but both genetic and environmental factors are believed to be involved. Management of the disease has greatly improved in recent years due to advances in pharmacologic treatment options (especially with new biologic agents) and the prognosis for patients is better than ever before. However, none of the available drugs has a curative potential. This review provides an overview on the classification and the clinical symptoms of the defined subgroups of JIA as well as pharmacotherapies for it. ***Conclusions:*** Treatment of children with JIA is challenging and complex. Since lengthy therapy might be necessary, a multidisciplinary pediatric rheumatology team is crucial for optimal treatment. Although a cure is unknown at this time, adequate treatment aims to preserve function of the joints as well as normal childhood development.

Introduction

The term juvenile idiopathic arthritis (JIA) comprises a heterogeneous group of several disease subtypes that are characterized by arthritis beginning before the age of 16 years with symptoms persisting for more than 6 weeks. All subtypes of JIA are of unknown causes. Although disease pathogenesis is most likely different for each of the respective subtypes, JIA is generally regarded as an autoimmune disease with the possible exception of systemic JIA. A combination of environmental (e.g., infectious) factors and a certain immunogenetic (e.g., specific HLA alleles) susceptibility may contribute to the disease. Since there is no pathognomonic finding for these disorders, diagnosis is based on the combined evaluation of medical history, clinical presentation and, to some extent, laboratory abnormalities.

The current classification was compiled by the International League of Associations for Rheumatology (ILAR). The previous terms of 'juvenile chronic arthritis' or 'juvenile rheumatoid arthritis', used in Europe or North America, respectively, were replaced by the term JIA [1]. Further classification into homogeneous subtypes allows for a better understanding of the pathogenesis and epidemiology as well as an improvement in the quality of international clinical studies.

KARGER

Fax +41 61 306 12 34
E-Mail karger@karger.ch
www.karger.com

0301–0163/09/0727–0004$26.00/0

Accessible online at:
www.karger.com/hre

Günther E. Dannecker
Department of Pediatric Rheumatology
Olgahospital Klinikum, DE–70176 Stuttgart (Gemany)
Tel. +49 711 278 72410, Fax +49 711 278 72419
E-Mail g.dannecker@klinikum-stuttgart.de

Table 1. Classification of juvenile idiopathic arthritis

Category	Definition
Systemic arthritis	Fever of at least 2 weeks' duration (daily for at least 3 days) and arthritis in ≥1 joint, plus one or more of the following: Erythematous rash Generalized lymph node enlargement Hepatomegaly and/or splenomegaly Serositis Exclusions: a, b, c, d
Oligoarthritis	Arthritis affecting ≤4 joints during the first 6 months of disease. There are 2 subcategories: Persistent = affecting ≤4 joints throughout the disease Extended = affecting >4 joints after the first 6 months of disease Exclusions: a, b, c, d, e
Polyarthritis, RF^-	Arthritis affecting ≥5 joints during the first 6 months of disease, RF negative. Exclusions: a, b, c, d, e
Polyarthritis, RF^+	Arthritis affecting ≥5 joints during the first 6 months of disease, RF positive at least 2 × on tests at least 3 months apart. Exclusions: a, b, c, e
Psoriatic arthritis	Arthritis + psoriasis or arthritis and at least two of the following: Dactylitis Nail pitting or onycholysis Psoriasis in a first-degree relative Exclusions: b, c, d, e
Enthesitis-related arthritis	Arthritis + enthesitis or arthritis or enthesitis with at least two of the following: Presence/history of sacroiliac joint tenderness and/or inflammatory lumbosacral pain $HLA\text{-}B27^+$ Onset of arthritis in a male over 6 years of age Acute (symptomatic) anterior uveitis History of ankylosing spondylitis, enthesitis-related arthritis, sacroiliitis with inflammatory bowel disease or acute anterior uveitis in a first-degree relative Exclusions: a, d, e
Undifferentiated arthritis	Arthritis that fulfills criteria in no category or in two or more of the above categories.

One of the major aims of the ILAR classification is the mutual exclusivity of the subtypes. Therefore, the following list of possible exclusions for each category was defined:

(a) Psoriasis or a history of psoriasis in the patient or first-degree relative.
(b) Arthritis in an HLA-B27-positive male beginning after the sixth birthday.
(c) Ankylosing spondylitis, enthesitis-related arthritis, sacroiliitis with inflammatory bowel disease or acute anterior uveitis or a history of one of these disorders in a first-degree relative.
(d) The presence of IgM rheumatoid factor and at least two occasions at least 3 months apart.
(e) The presence of systemic JIA in the patient.

RF = Rheumatoid factor.

Adapted from Petty et al. [1].

Classification

As noted, JIA is defined as arthritis of unknown etiology beginning before the age of 16 years and persisting for at least 6 weeks; other known conditions are excluded. As a consequence of the definition, JIA cannot be diagnosed before 6 weeks' duration; the final classification into one of the seven subgroups is usually done after 6 months [1]. The current categories of JIA are shown in table 1 [1], and the major epidemiologic features are listed in table 2 (modified according to Minden [2]).

Table 2. Major characteristics of juvenile idiopathic arthritis (JIA) and its categories

Category	Percentage of all JIA	Female %	Onset of disease years	ANAs %	HLA-B27+ %	Uveitis %
Systemic arthritis	6	50	5	14	5	1
Oligoarthritis	52	69	4	60	12	17
Polyarthritis, RF^-	13	76	7	35	12	5
Polyarthritis, RF^+	2	83	12	35	9	3
Psoriatic arthritis	8	64	7	41	20	10
Enthesitis-related arthritis	12	30	10	19	66	7
Undifferentiated	8	64	9	31	35	11
JIA total	100	64	6	46	22	12

Data are from the German Registry for Juvenile Arthritis (n = 3,510). ANAs = Antinuclear antibodies; RF = rheumatoid factor. Translated from Minden et al. [2].

The annual incidence of JIA is approximately 10 per 100,000 children among white children younger than 16 years old. Subtype distribution varies between countries. Whereas oligoarthritis is the most common subtype in Europe, its occurrence is less frequent in India and New Zealand, where polyarthritis is more common [3, 4]. Definitions and major characteristics of each subtype are presented in table 1 and table 2.

Systemic Arthritis

The clinical manifestation of JIA is dependent on the subtype. It is likely that some of the different subtypes represent different diseases with different causes; however, all result in joint inflammation. In 1897, Sir George Frederik Still published his observations of children with a systemic form of arthritis characterized by the classic triad of remittent fever, typical rash and arthritis [5]. More recently, systemic JIA has been speculated to belong to the autoinflammatory syndromes rather than to the group of autoimmune diseases. In the inflammatory process, two cytokines in particular, interleukin-1 (IL-1) and IL-6, play important roles [6, 7].

The systemic signs of fever and rash can precede the arthritis for weeks or even months. For a clear diagnosis, the presence of arthritis is necessary, accompanied or preceded by quotidian fever lasting at least 2 weeks with one or more of the signs listed in table 1. The febrile episodes are often accompanied by a characteristic macular, salmon-colored rash. The transient lesions are distributed most commonly over the trunk, are less than 10 mm in size and are usually nonpruritic. A possibly dangerous complication of systemic JIA is macrophage activation syndrome (MAS), whereby an uncontrolled activation of macrophages leads to haemophagocytosis [8]. Arthritis can initially be oligoarticular, but with persistence can result in the more severe polyarticular form, resulting in pronounced disability.

Growth failure is a peculiar feature of systemic-onset JIA, at least during the active course of the disease. Even in the absence of corticosteroid treatment, these patients experience impaired growth velocity. Dysregulated IL-6 production is likely partly responsible for this [9].

Diagnosis of systemic JIA is always based on clinical observation, and the differential diagnosis usually includes all different causes of fever of unknown origin including viral and bacterial infections and septicaemia, malignancies, Kawasaki syndrome, rheumatic fever and connective tissue diseases. Laboratory evaluation reveals leuko- and granulocytosis, as well as thrombocytosis; erythrocyte sedimentation rate (ESR) and C-reactive protein levels are also elevated. However, if MAS develops, leukopenia and thrombopenia can occur accompanied by highly elevated levels of ferritin, lactate hydrogenase and D-dimers.

Oligoarthritis

Arthritis that affects four or fewer joints during the first 6 months of the disease is called oligoarthritis. Within this category are two subtypes: persistent oligoarthritis, which does not extend to more than four joints, and extended oligoarthritis, in which arthritis extends to more than four joints after 6 months [1]. Oligoarthritis is typically characterized by early onset, usually affecting children aged 2 to 3 years. The arthritis is asymmetric and predominantly involves the large joints of the lower extremities excluding the hip. The most frequently affected joints – in decreasing order – are the knees, ankles, elbows and wrists. In approximately one third of patients, only a single joint is affected at disease onset.

Oligoarthritis predominately affects females. Diagnosis can be difficult since the signs of joint pain and swelling are not always recognized, and small children may not verbalize their complaints. Children, rather, present with easy fatigability with either cessation or regression in development. Sequelae include morning stiffness with warmth, painful motion or resisting the full range of motion. Muscle atrophy of affected extremities combined with accelerated growth may occur. A child with unilateral gonarthritis typically presents with a discrepancy in leg length resulting in a flexion and outward rotation of the affected knee (fig. 1).

Acute-phase reactants are normal or moderately increased, but a high ESR can also occur. Antinuclear antibodies (ANAs) are detected in about 60% of patients. The presence of ANAs conveys a risk of iridocyclitis [10], an inflammation of the iris and ciliary body of the eye. Iridocyclitis affects approximately 30% of patients with oligoarthritis. Although iridocyclitis can precede arthritis, it usually manifests itself within the first few years after the onset of arthritis. Due to its insidious and often asymptomatic onset, children with JIA should be screened at regular intervals by slit-lamp examination.

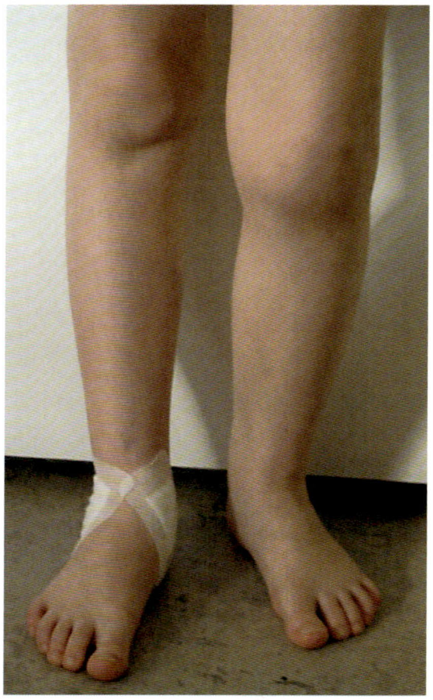

Fig. 1. Oligoarthritis affecting left knee and right ankle. Note flexion of left knee due to difference in leg length.

Rheumatoid Factor-Negative (RF^-) Polyarthritis

RF^- polyarthritis is defined as an arthritis that affects 5 or more joints during the first 6 months of the disease [1]. By definition, immunoglobulin-M rheumatoid factor (IgM-RF) is negative, and this subtype involves multiple large and small joints, very often in a symmetric fashion. The onset can be acute or insidious. Pain, confined movements and morning stiffness are the most prominent symptoms. Some patients with polyarthritis – especially those who are ANA positive – could be classified as having oligoarthritis, except that more joints are involved. Other patients present with only slight small joint swelling, but have pronounced stiffness and flexion contractions and a normal ESR. These patients are especially hard to diagnose.

Rheumatoid Factor-Positive (RF^+) Polyarthritis

This subtype is probably identical to the rheumatoid arthritis seen in adults. RF^+ polyarthritis occurs primarily in adolescent girls as a symmetric polyarthritis affecting the small joints of the hands and feet including the metacarpophalangeal, proximal interphalangeal and metatarsophalangeal joints. Rheumatoid nodules sometimes appear on the extensor surfaces of the elbows. By definition, the presence of IgM-RF is mandatory; however, anticyclic citrullinated peptide antibodies may also be of interest since they have been observed in adult patients with rheumatoid arthritis.

Enthesitis-Related Arthritis

This is the only subtype of JIA that affects more males than females, and it comprises approximately 10 to 15% of all patients with JIA. It is characterized by a combination of arthritis and enthesitis, which is defined as tenderness at the insertion of a tendon, ligament, joint capsule or fascia to the bone. Most patients express HLA-B27, long-known to be associated with arthritis; however, the etiology of enthesitis-related arthritis is still unknown [11].

Arthritis frequently affects the joints of the lower extremities, and the typical localization of the enthesitis is the calcaneal insertion of the Achilles tendon. Four or fewer joints are usually affected, but the disease can also take a polyarticular course. Involvement of the hip joint, an effect sometimes seen in this subgroup, can progress to include the sacroiliac joints and other joints of the axial skeleton, finally resulting in (juvenile) ankylosing spondylitis [12].

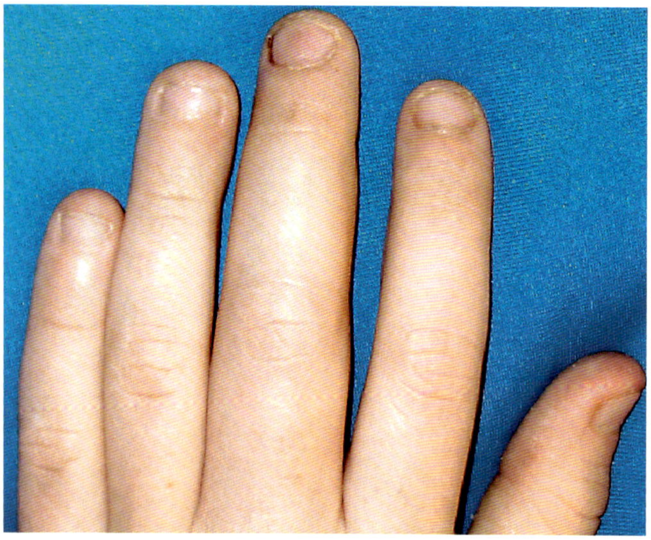

Fig. 2. Dactylitis of the middle finger.

Psoriatic Arthritis

Psoriatic arthritis is defined as arthritis with psoriasis or arthritis with two or more of the typical signs noted in table 1. In children, arthritis can precede psoriasis for many years. Often larger joints are affected in an asymmetric fashion, but small joints can also be affected. By definition, the presence of dactylitis (fig. 2), nail pitting, onycholysis or a positive family history supports the diagnosis; however, many children classified as having psoriatic arthritis according to the ILAR criteria might be better classified as having oligoarticular disease. Therefore, the definition of juvenile psoriatic arthritis is under scrutiny [12].

Undifferentiated Arthritis

This subgroup includes patients who do not fulfill the criteria of any of the other categories or who would fit into two or more subgroups. This category, therefore, does not represent a separate clinical subgroup.

Pharmacological Treatments

Treatment of children with JIA should focus not only on achieving optimal function of the joints, but also on preserving normal childhood development and minimizing negative impacts on the patient's family. Treatment of these patients is challenging and complex. Patients and their families may experience psychological problems, may need time to deal with all of the different aspects of therapy and may struggle financially.

Childhood rheumatic diseases are often neither benign nor short-lived [13]. Given the complex therapy that might be necessary for many years, a multidisciplinary pediatric rheumatology team is crucial for optimal treatment of these children. In addition to the pediatric rheumatologist, representatives from different specialties (e.g., an orthopedist, ophthalmologist, oral surgeon, physical and occupational therapists, social workers and psychologists) should be included as members of a cross-functional treatment team.

A combination of pharmacological interventions, physical therapy and psychosocial support is crucial in managing JIA. Because of space limitations, however, the focus here is on pharmacotherapy. Treatment should be aimed at complete control of the disease to prevent any long-term consequences, while being mindful of the possible side effects from therapy.

Although no drugs can cure JIA, treatment has changed dramatically within the last several years. Control of the disease can be achieved more effectively and much faster with fewer side effects. This encouraging development is due to great advances in pharmacologic options, especially the biologic agents.

Nonsteroidal Anti-Inflammatory Drugs (NSAIDs)

NSAIDs control pain and inflammation by inhibition of the enzyme cyclo-oxygenase (COX). Most of the NSAIDs used in children are nonselective, inhibiting COX-1 as well as COX-2; the latter is more responsible for promoting inflammation. NSAIDs have been the mainstay of therapy for many years and, for most children with JIA, are typically the first line of therapy. The most commonly used NSAIDs are naproxen and ibuprofen. With consistent application, response is usually seen in approximately 1 month. There is no significant difference between the available NSAIDs with respect to effectiveness; individual preferences include availability, experience and taste [14, 15]. With systemic-onset JIA, indomethacin (3 mg/kg/day) seems particularly effective. Although indomethacin is officially indicated for use in children over age 15 years, it is often used off-label in much younger patients. Most NSAIDs are well tolerated with few side effects in children (nausea, abdominal pain and decreased appetite). Mood changes and concentration difficulties can also occur and urine output should be monitored since these drugs can be nephrotoxic. A lesser-known side effect is the development of pseudoporphyria, especially induced by naproxen. Pseudoporphyria is characterized by flat hypopigmented scars in areas of minor skin trauma [16]. This side effect necessitates discontinuation of naproxen, as scars can persist for many years. Another NSAID, meloxicam, inhibits COX-1 as well as COX-2. It is given once daily and has been proven to be as effective and safe as naproxen [17].

Intra-Articular Steroid Injections

Intra-articular steroid injections are used as second-line treatment in children who have not responded to conventional NSAID therapy or as initial therapy in patients with oligoarthritis. Prior to initiation of injections, arthritis that is due to Lyme disease must be ruled out. Several studies have shown triamcinolone hexacetonide to be more effective than other preparations; therefore, it is the most widely used steroid for injection into the larger joints [18]. Response is usually seen within a few days after injection and a response rate of 60 to 70% is maintained for several months. This treatment can avoid or correct joint contractures and prevent the development of leg length discrepancy. Although not proven by scientific means, children seem to benefit from intensive physiotherapy and mild restriction in physical activity after injection therapy. Subcutaneous atrophy and hypopigmentation are frequent side effects of injections, especially in weight-bearing smaller joints (e.g., ankle, talocalcanear and talonavicular) [19–22].

Disease-Modifying Antirheumatic Drugs

Although intra-articular steroid injections result in an improvement in approximately two thirds to three fourths of patients, many children will have uncontrolled disease requiring more aggressive treatment.

Methotrexate (MTX)

MTX has become the second-line agent of choice for many children with persistent disease despite the combined use of NSAIDs, intra-articular corticosteroids and adequate physical therapy. In 1992, a randomized study demonstrated the efficacy of 10 mg/m^2 MTX once a week with 63% of patients demonstrating an improvement. The maximum effect of MTX is typically reached at a dose of 15 mg/m^2. The drug can be administered orally or by subcutaneous injection [23–25]. MTX is usually well tolerated; the most frequent side effects are liver enzyme elevations and gastrointestinal toxicities such as nausea and vomiting.

Sulfasalazine

Sulfasalazine can improve joint inflammation and laboratory parameters in children with JIA, especially in enthesitis-related arthritis. Long-term positive effects have been observed [26], but the rate of side effects is quite high (about 30%). Many patients discontinue treatment due to gastrointestinal toxicity and skin rashes. In patients with systemic-onset JIA, sulfasalazine and other drugs, e.g., gold salts, are contraindicated because they can trigger MAS.

Leflunomide

Leflunomide is a competitive inhibitor of the enzyme dihydro-orotate-dehydrogenase and inhibits de novo synthesis of pyrimidines. In adults with rheumatoid arthritis, the efficacy is similar to MTX. Experience in children is scarce. One comparison of MTX to leflunomide found that leflunomide was nearly as effective as MTX, and it was also effective in polyarthritic patients who either failed to respond to or could not tolerate MTX. The two drugs had comparable side effects [27].

Glucocorticoids

Glucocorticoids are very potent and fast-acting anti-inflammatory substances, but due to well-known side effects, systemic use should be restricted to patients with severe or life-threatening disease. A course of low-dose corticosteroids may be used to control pain and morning stiffness while patients are awaiting the therapeutic effects of MTX or another second-line agent ('bridging agent'). In severe cases, intravenous steroids (e.g., methylprednisolone) can be used alternatively in high doses (10–30 mg/kg/dose) for up to 3 days, resulting in an immediate profound, but short-lasting, anti-inflammatory effect.

Biologic Agents

The introduction of biologic medications, especially the arrival of the antitumor necrosis factors (TNFs), has dramatically improved the treatment of childhood rheumatic diseases. The efficacy of TNFs has been demonstrated in experimental and human arthritis models and the successful clinical application of TNF-blockers demonstrates the central role of this cytokine in the pathogenesis of JIA. Cytokine antagonists do, however, carry a risk of immunosuppression and data are scarce in regards to long-term safety. Therefore, at the present time, the use of biologic agents is typically restricted to patients who do not respond to conventional therapy or experience intolerable side effects from other drugs. Pediatric rheumatologists should carefully monitor therapy with biologic agents, including patient participation in appropriate long-term registries.

TNF-Blocking Agents

Etanercept is a soluble TNF-receptor fusion protein consisting of TNF-receptor monomers fused to the Fc domain of human IgG1. The fusion protein binds to TNF-α and TNF-β and inhibits interaction with the appropriate receptor. Other TNF-blocking agents are infliximab, a chimeric monoclonal anti-TNF antibody, and adalimumab, a recombinant completely humanized IgG1 anti-TNF antibody. The efficacy of etanercept has been demonstrated in a double-blind, placebo-controlled study in patients with polyarticular JIA [28]. The rapid efficacy and tolerable safety profile of etanercept have been confirmed by additional studies [29]. Etanercept is approved as an anti-TNF agent for pediatric use and is especially effective in patients with polyarticular disease, where a response rate of approximately 70% can be achieved. Etanercept and other anti-TNF agents are less effective in children with systemic JIA with a response rate of about 30% [29]. The efficacy of all three TNF-blocking agents is comparable [30–32]. Adalimumab has been recently approved for pediatric use in the United States for children aged 4 years and older and in Europe for children aged 13 and older. In children with severe, corticosteroid-dependent uveitis, either infliximab or adalimumab in combination with MTX may be effective [29].

Other Biologic Modifiers

Anakinra is a recombinant IL-1 receptor antagonist that works by inhibiting the proinflammatory mechanism of IL-1. Tocilizumab is a humanized anti-IL-6 receptor monoclonal antibody [33]. Both have shown some promising effects in patients with systemic JIA [7, 33]. Other anti-IL-1 inhibitors are being tested in patients with systemic JIA. Among these are rilonacept, an IL-1 receptor antagonist, and canakinumab, an anti-IL-1 monoclonal antibody. Both have much longer half-lives than anakinra, which must be administered as a daily subcutaneous injection. The often-painful injections are a major drawback of anakinra. Other biologic agents such as abatacept, a fusion protein consisting of a T-cell activating antigen and IgG1 [34], and rituximab, an anti-B-cell antibody [35], are being evaluated for use in children with JIA. Recently, abatacept was found to be a rational alternative treatment for children with JIA [34].

Growth Hormone Replacement Treatment

Patients with JIA who receive corticosteroid treatment for more than 1 year and exhibit abnormal growth velocity should be considered candidates for growth hormone replacement therapy [36].

Conclusions

JIA is an important cause of short-term and long-term disability and it should not be considered a benign disease. The course in an individual child is impossible to predict, but certain prognostic generalizations can be made. Children with oligoarthritis are at risk of developing uveitis, which can be a major prognostic complication. Otherwise, patients with oligoarthritis generally have the best outcome. However, even in these patients, the rate of remission after 10 years is still less than 50%. The outcome in polyarticular patients is much worse, especially in RF^+ polyarthritis where remission rates as low as 6% have been reported [37]. The outcome of systemic JIA is highly variable. Approximately 50% of patients have monocyclic or intermittent episodes of disease with a rather good prognosis. In patients with an unremitting course, systemic inflammation eventually resolves, but chronic arthritis with major and substantial joint destruction can evolve [38]. Despite the new biologic modifiers and, in some cases, drugs like thalidomide [39], patients with polyarticular or systemic JIA represent the most severe and challenging of all the subtypes.

Acknowledgment

The authors would like to thank Dr. A. Hospach for providing figures 1 and 2.

Disclosure Statement

G.E.D. declares membership on advisory committees or review panels for Wyeth, Pfizer and Bristol-Myers Squibb for which he has received honoraria. P.Q. declares no conflict of interest.

References

1 Petty RE, Southwood TR, Manners P, Baum J, Glass DN, Goldenberg J, He X, Maldonado-Cocco J, Orozco-Alcala J, Prieur AM, Suarez-Almazor ME, Woo P: International League of Associations for Rheumatology classification of juvenile idiopathic arthritis: second revision, Edmonton, 2001. J Rheumatol 2004;31:390–392.

2 Minden K: Epidemiologie; in Wagner N, Dannecker G (eds): Pädiatrische Rheumatologie. Heidelberg, Springer Medizin Verlag, 2007, pp 179–181.

3 Manners PJ, Bower C: Worldwide prevalence of juvenile arthritis why does it vary so much? J Rheumatol 2002;29:1520–1530.

4 Oen KG, Cheang M: Epidemiology of chronic arthritis in childhood. Semin Arthritis Rheum 1996;26:575–591.

5 Still G: On a form of chronic joint disease in children. Medico-Chirurgical Transactions 1897;80:47–59.

6 de Benedetti F, Martini A: Targeting the interleukin-6 receptor: a new treatment for systemic juvenile idiopathic arthritis? Arthritis Rheum 2005;52:687–693.

7 Pascual V, Allantaz F, Arce E, Punaro M, Banchereau J: Role of interleukin-1 (IL-1) in the pathogenesis of systemic onset juvenile idiopathic arthritis and clinical response to IL-1 blockade. J Exp Med 2005;201:1479–1486.

8 Behrens EM, Beukelman T, Paessler M, Cron RQ: Occult macrophage activation syndrome in patients with systemic juvenile idiopathic arthritis. J Rheumatol 2007;34: 1133–1138.

9 Souza LS, Machado SH, Brenol CV, Brenol JC, Xavier RM: Growth velocity and interleukin 6 concentrations in juvenile idiopathic arthritis. J Rheumatol 2008;35:2265–2271.

10 Ravelli A, Felici E, Magni-Manzoni S, Pistorio A, Novarini C, Bozzola E, Viola S, Martini A: Patients with antinuclear antibody-positive juvenile idiopathic arthritis constitute a homogeneous subgroup irrespective of the course of joint disease. Arthritis Rheum 2005;52:826–832.

11 Taurog JD: The mystery of HLA-B27: if it isn't one thing, it's another. Arthritis Rheum 2007;56:2478–2481.

12 Ravelli A, Martini A: Juvenile idiopathic arthritis. Lancet 2007;369:767–778.

13 Minden K, Niewerth M, Listing J, Biedermann T, Bollow M, Schontube M, Zink A: Long-term outcome in patients with juvenile idiopathic arthritis. Arthritis Rheum 2002; 46:2392–2401.

14 Giannini EH, Brewer EJ, Miller ML, Gibbas D, Passo MH, Hoyeraal HM, Bernstein B, Person DA, Fink CW, Sawyer LA, et al: Ibuprofen suspension in the treatment of juvenile rheumatoid arthritis. Pediatric Rheumatology Collaborative Study Group. J Pediatr 1990;117:645–652.

15 Leak AM, Richter MR, Clemens LE, Hall MA, Ansell BM: A crossover study of naproxen, diclofenac and tolmetin in seronegative juvenile chronic arthritis. Clin Exp Rheumatol 1998;6:157–160.

16 Schad SG, Kraus A, Haubitz I, Trcka J, Hamm H, Girschick HJ: Early onset pauciarticular arthritis is the major risk factor for naproxen-induced pseudoporphyria in juvenile idiopathic arthritis. Arthritis Res Ther 2007;9: R10.

17 Ruperto N, Nikishina I, Pachanov ED, Shachbazian Y, Prieur AM, Mouy R, Joos R, Zulian F, Schwarz R, Artamonova V, Emminger W, Bandeira M, Buoncompagni A, Foeldvari I, Falcini F, Baildam E, Kone-Paut I, Alessio M, Gerloni V, Lenhardt A, Martini A, Hanft G, Sigmund R, Simianer S: A randomized, double-blind clinical trial of two doses of meloxicam compared with naproxen in children with juvenile idiopathic arthritis: short- and long-term efficacy and safety results. Arthritis Rheum 2005;52: 563–572.

18 Eberhard BA, Sison MC, Gottlieb BS, Ilowite NT: Comparison of the intraarticular effectiveness of triamcinolone hexacetonide and triamcinolone acetonide in treatment of juvenile rheumatoid arthritis. J Rheumatol 2004;31:2507–2512.

19 Breit W, Frosch M, Meyer U, Heinecke A, Ganser G: A subgroup-specific evaluation of the efficacy of intraarticular triamcinolone hexacetonide in juvenile chronic arthritis. J Rheumatol 2000;27:2696–2702.

20 Padeh S, Passwell JH: Intraarticular corticosteroid injection in the management of children with chronic arthritis. Arthritis Rheum 1998;41:1210–1214.

21 Zulian F, Martini G, Gobber D, Plebani M, Zacchello F, Manners P: Triamcinolone acetonide and hexacetonide intra-articular treatment of symmetrical joints in juvenile idiopathic arthritis: a double-blind trial. Rheumatology (Oxford) 2004;43:1288–1291.

22 Sherry DD, Stein LD, Reed AM, Schanberg LE, Kredich DW: Prevention of leg length discrepancy in young children with pauciarticular juvenile rheumatoid arthritis by treatment with intraarticular steroids. Arthritis Rheum 1999;42:2330–2334.

23 Giannini EH, Brewer EJ, Kuzmina N, Shaikov A, Maximov A, Vorontsov I, Fink CW, Newman AJ, Cassidy JT, Zemel LS: Methotrexate in resistant juvenile rheumatoid arthritis. Results of the U.S.A.–U.S.S.R. double-blind, placebo-controlled trial. The Pediatric Rheumatology Collaborative Study Group and The Cooperative Children's Study Group. N Engl J Med 1992;326:1043–1049.

24 Ruperto N, Murray KJ, Gerloni V, Wulffraat N, de Oliveira SK, Falcini F, Dolezalova P, Alessio M, Burgos-Vargas R, Corona F, Vesely R, Foster H, Davidson J, Zulian F, Asplin L, Baildam E, Consuegra JG, Ozdogan H, Saurenmann R, Joos R, Pistorio A, Woo P, Martini A: A randomized trial of parenteral methotrexate comparing an intermediate dose with a higher dose in children with juvenile idiopathic arthritis who failed to respond to standard doses of methotrexate. Arthritis Rheum 2004;50:2191–2201.

25 Alsufyani K, Ortiz-Alvarez O, Cabral DA, Tucker LB, Petty RE, Malleson PN: The role of subcutaneous administration of methotrexate in children with juvenile idiopathic arthritis who have failed oral methotrexate. J Rheumatol 2004;31:179–182.

26 Van Rossum MA, van Soesbergen RM, Boers M, Zwinderman AH, Fiselier TJ, Franssen MJ, Ten Cate R, Van Suijlekom-Smit LW, Wulffraat NM, van Luijk WH, Oostveen JC, Kuis W, Dijkmans BA: Long-term outcome of juvenile idiopathic arthritis following a placebo controlled trial: sustained benefits of early sulfasalazine treatment. Ann Rheum Dis 2007;66:1518–1524.

27 Silverman E, Mouy R, Spiegel L, Jung LK, Saurenmann RK, Lahdenne P, Horneff G, Calvo I, Szer IS, Simpson K, Stewart JA, Strand V, the Leflunomide in Juvenile Rheumatoid Arthritis (JRA) Investigator Group: leflunomide or methotrexate for juvenile rheumatoid arthritis. N Engl J Med 2005; 352:1655–1666.

28 Lovell DJ, Giannini EH, Reiff A, Cawkwell GD, Silverman ED, Nocton JJ, Stein LD, Gedalia A, Ilowite NT, Wallace CA, Whitmore J, Finck BK: Etanercept in children with polyarticular juvenile rheumatoid arthritis. Pediatric Rheumatology Collaborative Study Group. N Engl J Med 2000;342: 763–769.

29 Horneff G, Schmeling H, Biedermann T, Foeldvari I, Ganser G, Girschick HJ, Hospach T, Huppertz HI, Keitzer R, Kuster RM, Michels H, Moebius D, Rogalski B, Thon A: The German Etanercept Registry for treatment of juvenile idiopathic arthritis. Ann Rheum Dis 2004;63:1638–1644.

30 Gerloni V, Pontikaki I, Gattinara M, Desiati F, Lupi E, Lurati A, Salmaso A, Fantini F: Efficacy of repeated intravenous infusions of an anti-tumor necrosis factor alpha monoclonal antibody, infliximab, in persistently active, refractory juvenile idiopathic arthritis: results of an open-label prospective study. Arthritis Rheum 2005;52:548–553.

31 Lovell D, Ruperto N, Goodman S, Reiff A, Martini A, Giannini E, Radin A, Rao V, Spencer-Grenn G: Preliminary data from the study of adalimumab in children with juvenile idiopathic arthritis. Arthritis Rheum 2004;50:S436.

32 Lahdenne P, Vahasalo P, Honkanen V: Infliximab or etanercept in the treatment of children with refractory juvenile idiopathic arthritis: an open label study. Ann Rheum Dis 2003;62:245–247.
33 Yokota S, Imagawa T, Mori M, Miyamae T, Aihara Y, Takei S, Iwata N, Umebayashi H, Murata T, Miyoshi M, Tomiita M, Nishimoto N, Kishimoto T: Efficacy and safety of tocilizumab in patients with systemic-onset juvenile idiopathic arthritis: a randomised, double-blind, placebo-controlled, withdrawal phase III trial. Lancet 2008;371:998–1006.
34 Ruperto N, Lovell DJ, Quartier P, Paz E, Rubio-Pérez N, Silva CA, Abud-Mendoza C, Burgos-Vargas R, Gerloni V, Melo-Gomes JA, Saad-Magalhães C, Sztajnbok F, Goldenstein-Schainberg C, Scheinberg M, Penades IC, Fischbach M, Orozco J, Hashkes PJ, Hom C, Jung L, Lepore L, Oliveira S, Wallace CA, Sigal LH, Block AJ, Covucci A, Martini A, Giannini EH; Paediatric Rheumatology International Trials Organization; Pediatric Rheumatology Collaborative Study Group: Abatacept in children with juvenile idiopathic arthritis: a randomised, double-blind, placebo-controlled withdrawal trial. Lancet 2008;372:383–391.
35 El-Hallak M, Binstadt BA, Leichtner AM, Bennett CM, Neufeld EJ, Fuhlbrigge RC, Zurakowski D, Sundel RP: Clinical effects and safety of rituximab for treatment of refractory pediatric autoimmune diseases. J Pediatr 2007;150:376–382.
36 Simon D, Prieur AM, Quartier P, Charles Ruiz J, Czernichow P: Early recombinant human growth hormone treatment in glucocorticoid-treated children with juvenile idiopathic arthritis: a 3-year randomized study. J Clin Endocrinol Metab 2007;92: 2567–2573.
37 Oen K, Malleson PN, Cabral DA, Rosenberg AM, Petty RE, Cheang M: Disease course and outcome of juvenile rheumatoid arthritis in a multicenter cohort. J Rheumatol 2002;29:1989–1999.
38 Singh-Grewal D, Schneider R, Bayer N, Feldman BM: Predictors of disease course and remission in systemic juvenile idiopathic arthritis: significance of early clinical and laboratory features. Arthritis Rheum 2006;54: 1595–1601.
39 Lehman TJ, Schechter SJ, Sundel RP, Oliveira SK, Huttenlocher A, Onel KB: Thalidomide for severe systemic onset juvenile rheumatoid arthritis: a multicenter study. J Pediatr 2004;145:856–857.

HORMONE
RESEARCH

Horm Res 2009;72(suppl 1):13–19
DOI: 10.1159/000229758

Published online: November 27, 2009

Natural History of Growth and Body Composition in Juvenile Idiopathic Arthritis

S. Bechtold[a] J. Roth[b]

[a]Division of Pediatric Endocrinology, University Children's Hospital, Munich, Germany; [b]Division of Pediatric Rheumatology, Children's Hospital of Eastern Ontario, University of Ottawa, Ottawa, Ont., Canada

Key Words
Juvenile idiopathic arthritis · Body composition

Abstract
Background: In patients with juvenile idiopathic arthritis (JIA), growth impairment and altered body composition, including disturbed skeletal development, are well-known long-term complications. Data on longitudinal growth in patients with systemic and polyarticular JIA reveal growth impairment in the active phases of the disease. With reduction in disease activity and lower glucocorticoid (GC) doses, some patients experience 'catch-up' growth; however, many have only a slight improvement in height standard deviation during puberty or after cessation of GC treatment. The consequence is a final height below the 3rd percentile and below the genetic height potential. Although few studies have specifically addressed body composition in children with JIA, studies on the development of bone mass have described notable deficits in both GC-treated and GC-naïve children. In recent years, the deficits in bone mass have been related, in part, to the deficits in muscle mass, which are prevalent in these patients. ***Conclusions:*** The major goal for physicians caring for patients with JIA is optimal disease control while maintaining normal growth. Early recognition of patients who develop prolonged growth disturbances and altered body composition is important as these abnormalities contribute to long-term morbidity and need to be addressed both diagnostically and therapeutically when treating children with JIA.

Introduction

Growth impairment and altered body composition, including disturbed bone development, are well-known complications over the long term in patients with juvenile idiopathic arthritis (JIA). Patients with the polyarticular and systemic forms of JIA are particularly affected. Both inflammatory cytokines and glucocorticoids (GCs) – by interfering with the growth hormone (GH)-insulin-like growth factor axis – are thought to be responsible for the delayed growth and altered body composition. Changes in resting energy expenditure and reduced dietary intake may further contribute. This article presents an overview of the natural course of growth and body composition in patients with JIA.

KARGER

Fax +41 61 306 12 34
E-Mail karger@karger.ch
www.karger.com

0301–0163/09/0727–0013$26.00/0

Accessible online at:
www.karger.com/hre

S. Bechtold
Division of Pediatric Endocrinology, University Children's Hospital
Lindwurmstr. 4, DE–80337 Munich (Germany)
Tel. +49 89 5160 2811, Fax +49 89 5160 4784
E-Mail susanne.bechtold@med.uni-muenchen.de

Growth in Patients with JIA

Disturbed linear growth occurs frequently in children with JIA, and its likelihood increases in children with systemic or polyarticular forms of the disease and with lengthy duration. Recognition of growth impairment is important because reduced final height is a permanent consequence of JIA, affecting 10–20% of these patients [1]. Although the precise etiology of growth retardation is unknown, multiple factors have been implicated. Sequelae of the disease itself, including elevated levels of proinflammatory cytokines, immobilization, catabolic imbalance and food deprivation with malnutrition, may be contributory. In addition, growth may be hampered by administration of GCs, an often necessary treatment [2].

When Sir G.F. Still first described systemic JIA in 1897, he noted a general arrest of growth when the disease began in early childhood [3]. In 1956, Ansell and Bywaters, reporting on growth retardation in 119 children with JIA, noted that disease activity and the use of GCs were the main causes of growth disturbance [4]. Even in the absence of treatment with GCs, however, growth retardation has been observed. Data from a longitudinal study conducted over 4.9 ± 2.8 years (until near final height) revealed a correlation between disease subtype, disease duration and severity and growth development. Patients with systemic JIA lost 0.55 height standard deviation score (SDS) and patients with polyarticular JIA lost 0.7 height SDS during the observation period [5]. More recently, in patients with systemic JIA followed for more than 9 years, Liem and Rosenberg reported a mean decrease in height SD from +0.4 to –1.8 SD, with the height loss starting 2 years after disease onset [6].

Short Stature in Adulthood

How many patients with JIA have short stature in adulthood? Retrospective final height data from a registry of 65 patients showed that nearly 11% of patients with JIA had a final height below the 3rd percentile. All of these patients had polyarticular disease. Predisposing factors included the use of systemic GCs and prolonged disease activity. If GC therapy was necessary for more than 12 months, patients had a reduction in final height of 11.6 cm in relation to their target height [7].

A retrospective analysis of growth development in 24 patients with systemic JIA showed a mean height loss of 2.7 SD during GC treatment, which was positively correlated with the duration of therapy. After GC cessation, 70% of patients experienced 'catch-up' growth; however, mean final height was –2.0 SD and 87% of patients had a final height below their target height [1].

Bechtold et al. conducted a 4-year prospective study of GH treatment in patients with JIA, in which 20 patients (13 females, 7 males) who were not treated with GH served as the control group. Control subjects were initially prepubertal (mean age 9.6 ± 2.1 years) and received GCs and regular drug therapy as required by the disease state, including nonsteroidal anti-inflammatory drugs, slow-acting anti-inflammatory agents, methotrexate or cyclosporine A [8]. Their height SD decreased from –2.3 ± 1.3 to –3.0 ± 1.5 SD, and total height loss after 4 years expressed as height SDS was 0.7 SD. Five patients experienced stabilization or increase in height SD. Individual growth curves are shown in figure 1a (males) and figure 1b (females) for this group.

We obtained final height data for 18 of the control subjects (12 females, 6 males) from this study. All patients had systemic or polyarticular JIA. At disease onset, the mean age was 4.0 ± 2 years; at study start, the mean age was 10.1 ± 2 years; at final height, the mean age was 18.4 ± 1.4 years. At disease onset, the mean height was –0.4 ± 0.2 SD. Over the following years, these patients lost more than 3 SDs for height and had a mean height at the start of puberty of –3.49 ± 1.7 SD. Thereafter, there was a stabilization of height development with a mild increase of height SD during the pubertal years and a final height of –3.37 ± 2.0 SD (fig. 2). In relation to target height, patients lost 3.34 ± 2.4 SD. Only 4 of 18 patients (22%) reached a final height within their target height range. Multiple regression analyses revealed that the standardized height gain was most influenced by mean erythrocyte sedimentation rate, mean C-reactive protein level and mean prednisolone dose (cumulative R^2 with 0.67, $p < 0.05$) [9]. The tremendous height SDS loss during the prepubertal years in this patient group is comparable to retrospective data reported by Simon et al. [1]. Since patients in the aforementioned study were treated with lower doses of GCs, it is possible that the disease activity itself notably influenced growth development.

Growth in Patients with JIA: Conclusions

Based on current data, marked linear growth impairment is still a problem in about 10% of patients with JIA. Modern cytokine antagonists have positively affected height development, although not in all patients. In a study by Tynjälä et al., 10 of 36 patients (28%) with polyarticular or systemic JIA showed a delayed growth veloc-

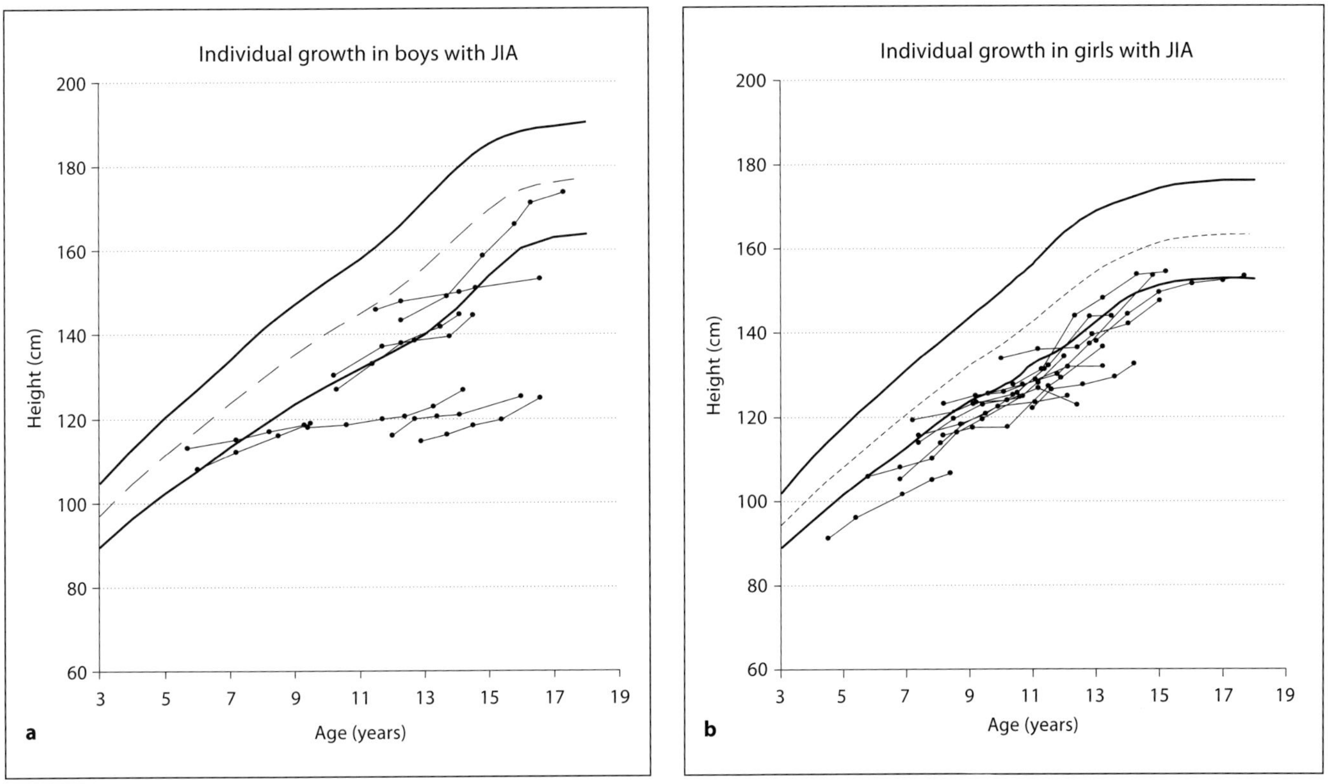

Fig. 1. Individual growth curves (•—•—•) in patients with juvenile idiopathic arthritis according to sex: **a** boys; **b** girls. Dashed lines represent the 50th percentile; uninterrupted lines represent the 3rd and 97th percentiles. Reference data from: Prader A, Largo RH, Molinari L, Issler C: Physical growth of Swiss children from birth to 20 years of age. First Zurich longitudinal study of growth and development. Helv Paediatr Acta 1989;52(suppl):1–125. (Reproduced with permission from Bechtold et al. [8]. ©2003, Elsevier.)

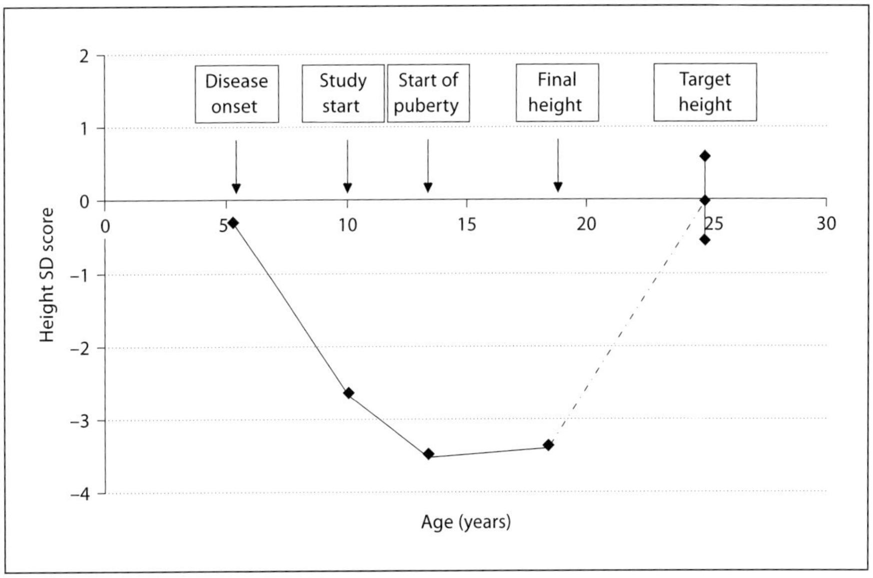

Fig. 2. Growth development and final height in relation to target height in patients with systemic and polyarticular juvenile idiopathic arthritis. SD = Standard deviation.

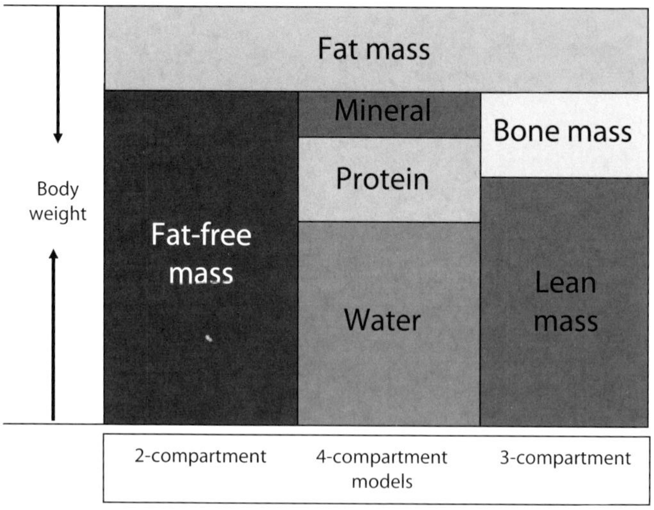

Fig. 3. Schematic representation of 2-, 3- and 4-compartment models of body composition.

ity both before and after antitumor necrosis factor treatment [10]. Thus, the major goal for the treating physician is optimal disease control while maintaining normal growth. In patients with JIA and reduced growth velocity, early intervention strategies may be warranted, and in this setting data from studies of early initiation of GH treatment are promising [11].

Body Composition in Patients with JIA

Abnormalities in body composition have been well documented in adults with rheumatoid arthritis (RA). The terms 'rheumatoid cachexia' and 'rheumatoid cachectic obesity' have been used to describe the sequelae of decreased lean body mass, increased fat mass (FM), reduced total energy expenditure and increased whole-body catabolism [12]. Cytokines are thought to play a major role in the development of this altered body composition. The resulting loss of muscle function and increased susceptibility to infections likely contribute significantly to disease-associated morbidity in patients with RA [12].

In patients with JIA, less is known about body composition effects because of the difficulties in assessing these parameters in growing children [13]. Despite the difficulty, alterations in body composition are of concern because they may impact long-term prognosis. As reviewed by Roth et al., recent evidence suggests that the accrual of bone mass depends largely on muscle mass and function [14]. In addition, muscle function is now recognized as critical for the preservation and restoration of joint function [15]. Increased FM may also convey increased cardiovascular risk. Thus, achieving and maintaining normal body composition will be a key end point for optimal treatment of patients with JIA.

Assessment of Body Composition

Direct measurement of body composition by chemical analysis is not possible in humans; therefore, various methods for indirect assessment have been developed. Techniques such as bioimpedance analysis, isotope dilution, hydrostatic weighing and skinfold thickness determination assess body composition using calculations based on equations obtained in certain populations. Unfortunately, these calculations might not be applicable or accurate when evaluating certain patient populations. For proper assessment of body composition, FM, lean body mass and bone mass need to be measured. Traditional methods rely mainly on a 2-component model that measures FM and fat-free mass (FFM) (fig. 3). [13]. Newer methods that also measure 2 components, e.g., isotope dilution techniques, bioimpedance analysis and hydrostatic weighing, have been developed. Since the 2-component models rely on assumptions of constant composition of FM and FFM, their accuracy has recently been questioned in both growing children and certain disease states [13].

Absorptiometric methods using the different absorption characteristics of X-rays at discrete wavelengths offer a more objective assessment and also allow for a multicompartment assessment of FM, muscle mass and bone mass. Each of these compartments must be separately assessed to determine long-term morbidity, analyze pathogenetic mechanisms and monitor therapeutic interventions.

To our knowledge, no studies have specifically addressed body composition in patients with JIA. Instead, most studies have assessed bone mass using dual energy X-ray absorptiometry (DXA) or peripheral quantitative computed tomography (pQCT). While DXA does have technical limitations and pitfalls, whole-body DXA scans are useful and pQCT might be of particular use in longitudinal studies in JIA.

DXA

Whole-body DXA scans can be performed on children and allow for the separate analysis of whole-body bone mass, fat mass and lean mass. It must be noted that, as a 2-dimensional measurement method, DXA is dependent on body size. Therefore, results must be corrected for height in children with growth retardation [14]. This may be more relevant for the determination of absolute values of each compartment in relation to normative data (z-scores) and less so for the relationship and percentage of each compartment.

pQCT

Most recently, QCT (especially pQCT) has gained a role in assessing bone density and geometry. This 3-dimensional technique collects measurements on the radius or the tibia and also of muscle cross-sectional area (CSA) and fat area separately from bone area. Since normative data for each compartment have been established, body composition can be assessed by pQCT. A disadvantage is that measurements at the extremities do not necessarily reflect total body composition. Nevertheless, pQCT might prove especially useful in the longitudinal assessment of each of the compartments in response to treatment [16].

Role of Glucocorticoids on Body Composition

Cross-sectional studies have shown that GC administration contributes to decreased bone mass at the femur and the spine, a reduction only partly explained by a decrease in body height [17]. In one study, patients with JIA who were receiving GC therapy had reduced bone mass at the spine compared with patients receiving nonsteroidal anti-inflammatory drugs [18]. There was no difference between the two groups with regards to calcium or vitamin D intake or serum levels [18]. In general, nearly all pediatric arthritis studies involve a small number of patients and heterogeneity in the amount and duration of GC treatment. GCs can induce growth retardation and thus must be corrected for to avoid false-low results in any evaluation. Lastly, the severity of the disease correlates with the likelihood of treatment with GCs, making it difficult to ascertain whether these effects are due to the inflammatory nature of JIA itself or the sequelae of GC therapy.

Critical Appraisal

No longitudinal studies on resting energy expenditure (REE) are available in patients with JIA, but one study has assessed REE in a cross-sectional sample using indirect calorimetry [19]. Knops et al. found markedly increased REE only in patients with systemic JIA who also had growth retardation and decreased FFM [19].

In cross-sectional studies, most of which used DXA scans, patients with all forms of JIA showed a marked decrease in bone mass at the spine and the peripheral skeleton [20]. Bone mass may also be reduced in patients who experience growth retardation, but this finding is not as clear-cut as many of these studies did not correct for results for body height. Other findings of interest are that bone mass was lower in patients with polyarticular disease compared with oligoarticular disease and that calcium and vitamin D intake was similar in both groups and did not correlate with variables of bone metabolism [20, 21]. In contrast, muscle mass and bone mass correlated highly [20]. In studies of GC-naïve patients, 30% of prepubertal children and a similar percentage of postpubertal girls had decreases in whole body bone mass (z-score <-1) [22, 23]. According to a multiple regression analysis, 75% of the variation in bone mass could be explained by changes in muscle mass [22, 23]. It was particularly interesting that patients with JIA experienced a severe decrease in bone mass despite the fact that 33% of patients in these two studies did not have active arthritis at the time of measurement.

Studies using pQCT show that children in all subgroups of JIA have significant ($p < 0.05$) bone loss. Trabecular bone density next to inflamed joints was particularly affected, whereas cortical bone density was normal. The main changes were decreases in cortical thickness, muscle CSA and muscle force [24, 25]. In longitudinal studies, periosteal expansion has been observed. Although this results in some increase in bone strength, it clearly represents a pathologic geometric structure of diaphyseal bone in the developing skeleton [26].

A recent study using pQCT of the tibia in patients with JIA has shown that, while both muscle CSA and parameters of bone geometry were decreased compared with those in healthy children, the reductions in bone mass and geometry for a given reduction in muscle CSA were more than would be expected versus measurements in healthy children [27]. Thus, while considerable bone loss might occur secondarily to the loss of muscle mass, an interaction of inflammatory cytokines and medication may exacerbate deficits of bone mass independently.

Longitudinal Studies and Outcomes

Lien et al. conducted a 2-year longitudinal study in patients with JIA and healthy control subjects using whole-body DXA scans [28]. Significant differences were noted in total body bone mineral content (35 g less in patients with JIA [95% CI 2–68; $p < 0.035$]); total lean body mass (1.2 kg less in patients with JIA [95% CI 0.5–1.8; $p < 0.001$]), and percentage of total body fat (2.8% greater in patients with JIA [95% CI 1.2–4.4; $p < 0.001$]) [28]. Up to 50% of adults with a history of JIA experience decreased bone mass. Predictors include ongoing disease activity, long-term GC treatment and polyarticular disease course [29, 30]. One long-term outcome study in young adults with a history of JIA found that those patients with low bone mass also had low lean body mass [30]. However, the results were difficult to interpret since patients with low bone and lean body mass were also much shorter than those with normal values, and the investigators did not correct for height. These results may, therefore, be more reflective of growth delay than true reductions in bone and lean body mass.

Conclusions

Patients with JIA show decreased bone and muscle mass and increased FM. These findings are similar to the abnormalities observed in adults with RA. The reduction in bone mass may represent secondary bone loss or a failure to accrue bone mass. Existing data suggest that a decrease in muscle mass and force is a major contributing factor to the deficits in bone mass. The decrease in muscle mass can largely be explained by atrophy that is due either to general inactivity or to local bone and joint lesions limiting the range of motion. In addition, the direct actions of cytokines and medication, such as GCs, on muscle and bone must be considered. Increased REE may also be present in certain patient subgroups. All of these findings contribute substantially to long-term morbidity and need to be addressed both diagnostically and therapeutically when treating children with JIA. Additional prospective studies are required to precisely define the extent of the problem as well as its timing in relation to disease activity.

Disclosure Statement

S.B. declares no conflict of interest. J.R. received speaker's fees from Amgen and Schering and honoraria from Roche.

References

1 Simon D, Fernando C, Czernichow P, Prieur AM: Linear growth and final height in patients with systemic juvenile idiopathic arthritis treated with longterm glucocorticoids. J Rheumatol 2002;29:1296–1300.
2 Kotaniemi A: Growth retardation and bone loss as determinations of axial osteopenia in juvenile chronic arthritis. Scand J Rheumatol 1997;26:14–18.
3 Still GF: On a form of chronic joint disease in children. Am J Dis Child 1978;132:195–200 [reprinted from Medico-Chirurgical Transactions, 1897, vol 80].
4 Ansell BM, Bywaters EG: Growth in Still's disease. Ann Rheum Dis 1956;15:295–319.
5 Polito C, Strano CG, Olivieri AN, Alessio M, Iammarrone CS, Todisco N, Papale MR: Growth retardation in non-steroid treated juvenile rheumatoid arthritis. Scand J Rheumatol 1997;26:99–103.
6 Liem JJ, Rosenberg AM: Growth pattern in juvenile rheumatoid arthritis. Clin Exp Rheumatol 2003;21:663–668.
7 Zak M, Müller J, Karup Pedersen F: Final height, armspan, subischial leg length and body proportions in juvenile chronic arthritis. A long-term follow-up study. Horm Res 1999;52:80–85.
8 Bechtold S, Ripperger P, Häfner R, Said E, Schwarz HP: Growth hormone improves height in patients with juvenile idiopathic arthritis: 4-year data of a controlled study. J Pediatr 2003;143:512–519.

9 Bechtold S, Ripperger P, Dalla Pozza R, Bonfig W, Häfner R, Michels H, Schwarz HP: Growth hormone increases final height in patients with juvenile idiopathic arthritis: data from a randomized controlled study. J Clin Endocrinol Metab 2007;92:3013–3018.
10 Tynjälä P, Lahdenne P, Vähäsalo P, Kautiainen H, Honkanen V: Impact of anti-TNF treatment on growth in severe juvenile idiopathic arthritis. Ann Rheum Dis 2006;65: 1044–1049.
11 Simon D, Prieur AM, Quartier P, Charles Ruiz J, Czernichow P: Early recombinant human growth hormone treatment in glucocorticoid-treated children with juvenile idiopathic arthritis: a 3-year randomized study. J Clin Endocrinol Metab 2007;92: 2567–2573.
12 Rall LC, Roubenoff R: Rheumatoid cachexia: metabolic abnormalities, mechanisms and interventions. Rheumatology (Oxford) 2004; 43:1219–1223.
13 Reilly JP: Assessment of body composition in infants and children. Nutrition 1998;14:821–825.
14 Roth J, Bechtold S, Borte G, Dressler F, Girschick H, Borte M: Osteoporosis in juvenile idiopathic arthritis – a practical approach to diagnosis and therapy. Eur J Pediatr 2007;166:775–784.
15 Herzog W, Longino D, Clark A: The role of muscles in joint adaptation and degeneration. Langenbecks Arch Surg 2003;388:305–315.
16 Bechtold S, Ripperger P, Bonfig W, Pozza RD, Haefner R, Schwarz HP: Growth hormone changes bone geometry and body composition in patients with juvenile idiopathic arthritis requiring glucocorticoid treatment: a controlled study using peripheral quantitative computed tomography. J Clin Endocrinol Metab 2005;90:3168–3173.
17 Kotaniemi A, Savolainen A, Kautiainen H, Kroeger H: Estimation of central osteopenia in children with chronic polyarthritis treated with glucocorticoids. Pediatrics 1993;91: 1127–1130.
18 Falcini F, Trapani S, Civinini R, Capone A, Ermini M, Bartolozzi G: The primary role of steroids on the osteoporosis in juvenile rheumatoid arthritis patients evaluated by dual energy x-ray absorptiometry. J Endocrinol Invest 1996;9:165–169.
19 Knops N, Wulffraat N, Lodder S, Houwen R, de Meer K: Resting energy expenditure and nutritional status in children with juvenile rheumatoid arthritis. J Rheumatol 1999;26: 2039–2043.
20 Pepmueller PH, Cassidy JT, Allen SH, Hillman LS: Bone mineralization and bone mineral metabolism in children with juvenile rheumatoid arthritis. Arthritis Rheum 1996; 39:746–757.
21 Kotaniemi A, Savolainen A, Kroger H, Kautiainen H, Isomaki H: Weight-bearing physical activity, calcium intake, systemic glucocorticoids, chronic inflammation and body constitution as determinants of lumbar and femoral bone mineral in juvenile chronic arthritis. Scand J Rheumatol 1999;28:19–26.
22 Henderson CJ, Cawkwell GD, Specker BL, Sierra RI, Wilmott RW, Campaigne BN, Lovell DJ: Predictors of total body bone mineral density in non-corticosteroid treated prepubertal children with juvenile rheumatoid arthritis. Arthritis Rheum 1997;40: 1967–1975.
23 Henderson CJ, Specker BL, Sierra RI, Campaigne BN, Lovell DJ: Total body bone mineral content in non-corticosteroid treated postpubertal females with juvenile rheumatoid arthritis. Arthritis Rheum 2000;43:531–540.
24 Bechtold S, Ripperger P, Dalla Pozza R, Schmidt H, Hafner R, Schwarz HP: Musculoskeletal and functional muscle-bone analysis in children with rheumatic disease using peripheral quantitative computed tomography. Osteoporosis Int 2005;16:757–763.
25 Roth J, Palm C, Scheunemann I, Ranke MB, Schweizer R, Dannecker GE: Musculoskeletal abnormalities of the forearm in patients with juvenile idiopathic arthritis relate mainly to bone geometry. Arthritis Rheum 2004;50:1277–1285.
26 Roth J, Linge M, Tzaribachev N, Schweizer R, Kuemmerle-Deschner J: Muskuloskeletal system in juvenile arthritis – a 4-year longitudinal study. Rheumatology (Oxford) 2007; 46:1180–1184.
27 Burnham JM, Shults J, Dubner SE, Sembhi H, Zemel BS, Leonard MB: Bone density, structure, and strength in juvenile idiopathic arthritis: importance of disease severity and muscle deficits. Arthritis Rheum 2008; 58:2518–2527.
28 Lien G, Selvaag AM, Flatø B, Haugen M, Vinje O, Sørskaar D, Dale K, Egeland T, Førre Ø: A two-year prospective controlled study of bone mass and bone turnover in children with early juvenile idiopathic arthritis. Arthritis Rheum 2005;52:833–840.
29 Zak M, Hassager C, Lovell DJ, Nielsen S, Henderson CJ, Pedersen FK: Assessment of bone mineral density in adults with a history of juvenile chronic arthritis: a cross-sectional long-term followup study. Arthritis Rheum 1999;42:790–798.
30 Lien G, Flatø B, Haugen M, Vinje O, Sørskaar D, Dale K, Johnston V, Egeland T, Førre Ø: Frequency of osteopenia in adolescents with early-onset juvenile idiopathic arthritis: a long-term outcome study of one hundred five patients. Arthritis Rheum 2003;48: 2214–2223.

HORMONE
RESEARCH

Horm Res 2009;72(suppl 1):20–25
DOI: 10.1159/000229759

Published online: November 27, 2009

Adult Outcomes of Patients with Juvenile Idiopathic Arthritis

Kirsten Minden

Children's University Hospital Charité Berlin and Epidemiology Unit, German Rheumatism Research Centre, Berlin, Germany

Key Words
Juvenile idiopathic arthritis · Outcome · Bone · Growth failure

Abstract
Background: Knowledge of the long-term outcomes of patients with juvenile idiopathic arthritis (JIA) has evolved during the past decade. Recent studies, using standardized classification criteria, new and reliable outcome measures and improved methods of statistical analyses, show that outcomes are still less than ideal. Approximately half of all young adults with JIA have ongoing active disease and over one third experience detectable degrees of disability and organ damage. These patients also show a distinctive pattern of growth disturbances. Most patients with general growth failure have systemic or polyarticular disease: significant short stature (final height standard deviation score <–2) has been noted in 41% of patients with systemic JIA and in 11% of patients with polyarticular JIA. In contrast, localized growth disturbances can be seen in patients with oligoarthritis. ***Conclusions:*** Despite its name, JIA can be a lifelong disorder. With early and more widespread use of biological and other innovative therapies, however, outcomes for patients with JIA should improve further.

Introduction

Juvenile idiopathic arthritis (JIA) is a common chronic disease and an important cause of acquired impairment and disability in children and adolescents. Research into the long-term outcome of patients with JIA has accumulated during the last 13 years, with at least ten large studies published. These studies, which were retrospective or cross-sectional, yielded varying results owing to the heterogeneity of the populations studied, the different classification criteria and assessment tools used and the differences in follow-up duration [1–10]. Nevertheless, all studies consistently showed that JIA is associated with increased mortality, significant morbidity from articular and extra-articular manifestations (e.g., growth disturbances, osteopenia and osteoporosis and vision loss), chronic disability and restricted participation in normal social activities. These recent results disprove the former belief that as many as 80% of children with JIA could expect to be free of inflammation by adulthood [11].

This review summarizes the most significant problems observed in patients with JIA as they enter adulthood, with special attention given to the physiological consequences of the disease.

KARGER

Fax +41 61 306 12 34
E-Mail karger@karger.ch
www.karger.com

0301–0163/09/0727–0020$26.00/0

Accessible online at:
www.karger.com/hre

K. Minden
German Rheumatism Research Centre Berlin, Epidemiology Unit
Children's University Hospital Charité Berlin, Campus Virchow, SPZ-Rheumatology
Augustenburger Platz 1, DE–13353 Berlin (Germany)
Tel. +49 30 2846 0632, Fax, +49 30 2846 0626, E-Mail minden@drfz.de

Table 1. Recent outcome studies of juvenile idiopathic arthritis (JRA, JCA) with a follow-up of at least 10 years

Study (year, country)	Patients assessed n	Mean disease duration years	% of patients with active disease	functional limitations HAQ > 0	erosive joint changes
Peterson et al. (1997, US) [1]	44	25	66	39	NG
Ruperto et al. (1997, Italy, US) [2]	227	15	NG	42	NG
Zak and Pedersen (2000, Denmark) [3]	65	26	37	46	NG[a]
Oen et al. (2002, Canada) [4]	392	11 (median)	44	55	NG[c]
Minden et al. (2002, Germany) [5]	215	17 (median)	55	39	NG[b]
Packham and Hall (2002, UK) [6]	246	28	54	NG[d]	NG[e]
Flatø et al. (2003, Norway) [7]	268	15	50	36	24
Fantini et al. (2003, Italy) [8]	683	10	67	NG	NG
Foster et al. (2003, UK) [9]	82	21 (median)	39	NG[f]	NG[g]
Arkela-Kautiainen et al. (2005, Finland) [10]	123	16	65	NG	NG

JRA = Juvenile rheumatoid arthritis; JCA = juvenile chronic arthritis; HAQ = Health Assessment Questionnaire; NG = not given.
[a] 22% had JCA-related major surgical interventions; [b] 2% had joint replacements; [c] 7% had joint replacements, in >30% erosions of the hips, feet, wrists and shoulders [15]; [d] 3% had severe functional limitations (HAQ score ≥1.5); [e] 51% had joint replacements; [f] 55% had severe functional limitations (HAQ score ≥1.0); [g] 32% had joint replacements.

Physical Outcomes

On a physical level, the disease consequences of JIA are clinically measurable signs and symptoms. They comprise such outcome parameters as mortality, persistent disease activity and organ system damage, including growth disorders.

Mortality

As with adult-onset inflammatory rheumatic diseases, JIA is associated with shortened life expectancy. In a population-based study, French et al. found a roughly 4-fold increase in overall mortality in patients with JIA compared with the general population [12]. Thomas and colleagues estimated that the standardized mortality ratio (SMR) in women and men with JIA was 5 and 3, respectively [13]. These SMRs were twice as high as those calculated for men and women with rheumatoid arthritis (RA). Whether cardiovascular diseases, infections or hematopoietic malignancies contributed to the increased SMR, as observed in patients with RA, is unknown [13].

Morbidity

Morbidity in patients with JIA in adulthood results primarily from articular symptoms. Studies evaluating the outcomes of arthritis patients from North America and Europe over the last 13 years showed that active arthritis is present in approximately 40–70% of patients after disease duration of 10 to 28 years (table 1) [1–10]. Despite differences in the data examined and the methodologies applied, the rates of active disease in early adulthood were relatively similar: approximately half of all patients with JIA continue to have detectable inflammation in adulthood. This finding refutes the concept that JIA becomes less inflammatory and 'burns out' with time.

Because JIA is a heterogeneous disorder, there are substantial differences regarding the persistence of active disease among various subgroups. Using life table analyses, patients with oligoarthritis were found to have the highest projected remission rates at 10 years (approximately 50%), while remission rates were about 40% in patients with systemic-onset and 15% in patents with polyarticular JIA [4, 14].

The longer the disease is active, the higher the risk of joint destruction. After 10 years of disease duration, at least one in four patients has developed radiographic joint changes (e.g., erosions, joint space narrowing or total destruction), and the hips and wrists are the most vulnerable sites [7, 15]. The inflammation causes such severe joint damage that patients usually require prosthetic joint replacements, often at a young age. Results from various studies show that from 2–50% of 20- to 35-year-old patients with JIA have received endoprostheses [4–6, 9]. Patients with systemic-onset arthritis have the highest frequency of joint replacements and the hip is the most frequently replaced joint.

Table 2. Studies on final height in adults with juvenile idiopathic arthritis (JRA, JCA)

Study (year, country)	Patients assessed, n	Mean, age years	Mean final height SDS, z-score	Patients with reduced final height, %
Minden et al. (2002, Germany) [5]	215	23	NG	1.4, <3rd percentile
Packham and Hall (2002, UK) [6]	259	28	–1.09 women, –0.65 men	NG
Lovell and White (1990, US) [22]	NG	NG	NG	17, <5th percentile
Gäre et al. (1995, Sweden) [23]	124	18	NG	0, ≤–2 SD
Zak et al. (1999, Denmark) [24]	65	32	–0.25 (whole group)	11, ≤–2 SD

JRA = Juvenile rheumatic arthritis; JCA = juvenile chronic arthritis; NG = not given; SD = standard deviation.

Prolonged active disease may also impair the entire musculoskeletal system in young adults with JIA. In cross-sectional, case-controlled studies, reduced bone mineral content and density were reported in a substantial number of adults with JIA [16–19]. The frequency of osteopenia in these studies varied from 15–46% at the lumbar spine and/or femoral head; the frequency of osteoporosis was 0 to 9%. Of note, even patients with oligoarthritis and those who had never received corticosteroids were affected. Risk factors included ongoing disease activity, functional limitations, reduced level of physical activity, long corticosteroid exposure and poor nutritional status. Thus, even though the majority of adults with JIA will have normal bone mass, a large subset is osteopenic in adulthood, which places them at increased risk for future fractures and corresponding morbidity.

Another well-known and important consequence of JIA is growth failure. Local disturbances in growth occur primarily at sites of inflammation and can take the form of overgrowth or undergrowth. There is a tendency toward accelerated maturation of epiphyses, which can lead to increased leg length, or overcrowding and fusion of the joint in wrists and ankles. Well-recognized local growth disturbances include leg length inequality, mandibular micrognathia and shortening of fingers, forearms, toes and feet; however, there are few data on their degree and frequency in adults with JIA. Discrepancies in limb length and micrognathia occur in up to a quarter of adult patients [5, 6].

Generalized growth failure in patients with JIA occurs secondarily to prolonged severe disease aggravated by treatment with corticosteroids. Therefore, it is more likely to develop in patients with systemic and polyarticular JIA. Sir G.F. Still, the 'father of British pediatrics', first described short stature in patients with systemic arthritis in 1897 [20]. Growth failure continues to affect patients with JIA today. In 2002, Simon and colleagues [21] reported a mean final height standard deviation score (SDS) of –2.0 in 24 patients with systemic JIA; 41% of the patients had a height more than 2 SDs below the mean. In addition, 87% had final heights that were below target height based on midparental height. Additional studies reported short stature in 1–17% of adults with JIA (final height expressed as SDS or percentile calculated from normative population height data) (table 2) [5, 6, 22–24]. Although the percentage of JIA subjects with reduced final height has decreased over the last decade, clinicians are still confronted with the challenge of treating patients with JIA and retarded linear growth.

This is illustrated by data from the German pediatric rheumatologic database [K. Minden et al., unpublished data, 2005]. Although the average final linear height of 18-year-old women and men with JIA (165 and 176 cm, respectively) was similar to that of a reference group (166 and 179 cm, respectively), the distribution of height in the JIA group differed considerably (fig. 1). This finding suggests a systematic shift toward reduced height in the affected group. Patients with seronegative polyarthritis and systemic arthritis were predominantly affected. The average height SDS for women and men with seronegative polyarthritis was –0.47 and –0.57, respectively; for systemic arthritis, it was –0.5 and –2.07, respectively. Although these data must be interpreted with caution since the number of 18-year-olds included in the database was small, they underline the fact that final height will remain an important disease outcome parameter in JIA in the coming years.

Physical restrictions in young adults with JIA may also result from manifestations outside the musculoskeletal system. Among them, uveitis is one of the most common and threatening complications because of the risk of ocular morbidity and vision loss. Approximately 13% of patients develop uveitis, and one third of them will have significant vision loss from complications including cataracts, glaucoma and band keratopathy. Fortunately,

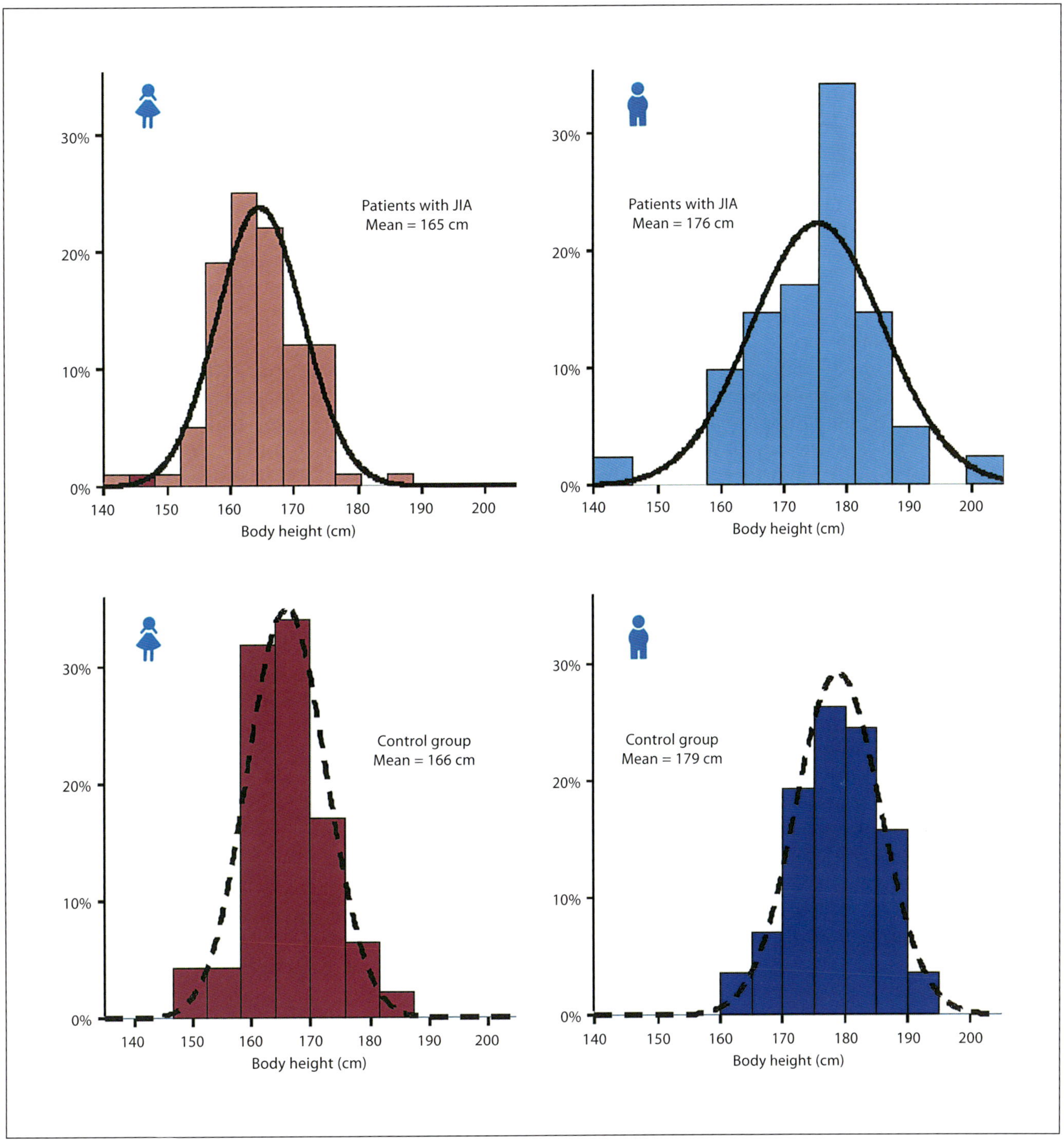

Fig. 1. Distribution of height in 18-year-old patients (100 women and 41 men) with JIA compared with control subjects (47 women and 57 men). Data from the German pediatric rheumatologic database, 2005, compared with data from the German Health Interview and Examination Survey for Children and Adolescents.

blindness due to uveitis is rare today, with a rate of <1% [25]. Data on other extra-articular sequelae are scarce. For example, longer follow-up studies are needed to clarify the risk of cardiovascular and lymphoproliferative disorders in these patients.

Overall, more than one third of young people with JIA will experience significant morbidity in adulthood, due to joint damage, growth disturbances, osteopenia and osteoporosis and extra-articular organ damage, such as vision loss.

Functional Outcomes

Despite the long-term persistence of disease activity in most patients, a pronounced improvement in functional outcome has been documented in the past decade. In the 1970s, the percentage of patients with no functional limitation (i.e., Steinbrocker functional class I) ranged from 25–40%. The percentage of patients with serious functional disability (Steinbrocker functional classes III and IV) ranged from 17–22%. By the 1990s, a higher percentage of patients without functional limitation (60%) and a lower percentage of patients with serious functional disability (10%) were observed. Most current outcome studies used not only the Steinbrocker functional classes to assess physical disability, but also a more sensitive measure of function, the Health Assessment Questionnaire (HAQ). The HAQ is a self-reported measure of function in performing activities of daily living and self-care. Its score ranges from 0 to 3 and an HAQ score of >1.0 indicates moderate to severe disability. Considering all patients with JIA, approximately 40% of young adults are somewhat limited in their functional capacity as assayed by the HAQ (table 1). Approximately 10% are in need of assistance to manage their daily routines, which is similar to the percentage of patients exhibiting serious disability according to the Steinbrocker functional class system. Severe disability is most frequently seen in patients with seropositive polyarthritis and systemic disease onset, followed by patients with seronegative polyarthritis and extended oligoarthritis. In contrast, patients with persistent oligoarthritis rarely exhibit functional disability in early adulthood [4, 5, 7].

Social Outcomes

Physical and functional restrictions may notably impact a person's ability to be a productive member of society. For many young people with JIA, entering the labor force, a main indicator of productivity, is difficult. Several studies noted lower employment rates for patients with JIA compared with age-matched local control subjects, despite comparable, if not better, academic achievement in patients with JIA. The lower employment rates were due primarily to higher unemployment [1, 6, 7, 9], extended training periods [5] or early retirement. Data from the German rheumatologic database indicate that employment rates in men and women with JIA remain lower than those in age-matched control subjects and even lower than those in patients with RA or adult-onset spondyloarthropathies [26].

The impact of JIA and its treatment on physical, functional and social outcomes is reflected in impaired patient health and perceived quality of life. Health in young adults with JIA has been repeatedly analyzed using quality-of-life measures, such as the Short Form 36 (SF 36). Its scores range from 0 to 100, with 0 representing the worst health and 100, the best. Using the SF 36, two controlled outcome studies showed that adults with JIA judged their quality of life as lower than that of age- and sex-matched control subjects. Young adults felt particularly impaired in their 'physical health' (e.g., physical functioning, vitality and pain) [1, 9]. Young people with active JIA reported a substantially lower quality of life than those who had achieved remission, which emphasizes the importance of an effective therapy with complete suppression of disease activity.

Conclusions

Recent outcome studies demonstrate that JIA can be a lifelong disorder despite its name. Approximately 10–20% of 20- to 35-year-old persons with JIA endure physical, functional and social restrictions. However, all studies reporting long-term prognosis included patients with disease onset in the 1960s to 1980s, when therapy differed from the current standard of care. Aggressive therapy with immunomodulating agents (i.e., biologics) is now the standard to effectively treat children with JIA. There is justified hope that new treatment approaches will result in marked improvements in long-term outcomes in patients with JIA.

Disclosure Statement

The author has received consulting and lecture fees from Abbott Laboratories, Wyeth Pharmaceuticals, Bristol-Myers Squibb, Merck and Pfizer.

References

1 Peterson LS, Mason T, Nelson AM, O'Fallon WM, Gabriel SE: Psychosocial outcomes and health status of adults who have had juvenile rheumatoid arthritis. Arthritis Rheum 1997; 12:2235–2240.

2 Ruperto N, Levinson JE, Ravelli A, Shear ES, Link Tague B, Murray K, Martini A, Giannini EH: Long-term health outcomes and quality of life in American and Italian inception cohorts of patients with juvenile rheumatoid arthritis. I. Outcome status. J Rheumatol 1997;24:945–951.

3 Zak M, Pedersen FK: Juvenile chronic arthritis into adulthood: a long-term follow-up study. Rheumatol 2000;38:198–204.

4 Oen K, Malleson PN, Cabral DA, Rosenberg AM, Petty RE, Cheang M: Disease course and outcome of juvenile rheumatoid arthritis in a multicenter cohort. J Rheumatol 2002;29:1989–1999.

5 Minden K, Niewerth M, Listing J, Biedermann T, Bollow M, Schöntube M, Zink A: Long-term outcome in patients with juvenile idiopathic arthritis. Arthritis Rheum 2002; 46:2392–2401.

6 Packham JC, Hall MA: Long-term follow-up of 246 adults with juvenile idiopathic arthritis: functional outcome. Rheumatology (Oxford) 2002;41:1428–1435.

7 Flatø B, Lien G, Smerdel A, Vinje O, Dale K, Johnston V, Sørskaar D, Moum T, Ploski R, Førre Ø: Prognostic factors in juvenile rheumatoid arthritis: a case-control study revealing early predictors and outcome after 14.9 years. J Rheumatol 2003;30:386–393.

8 Fantini F, Gerloni V, Gattinara M, Cimaz R, Arnoldi C, Lupi E: Remission in juvenile chronic arthritis: a cohort study of 683 consecutive cases with a mean 10 year followup. J Rheumatol 2003;30:579–584.

9 Foster HE, Marshall N, Myers A, Dunkley P, Griffiths ID: Outcome in adults with juvenile idiopathic arthritis: a quality of life study. Arthritis Rheum 2003;48:767–775.

10 Arkela-Kautiainen M, Haapasaari J, Kautiainen H, Vilkkumaa I, Mälkiä E, Leirisalo-Repo M: Favourable social functioning and health related quality of life of patients with JIA in early adulthood. Ann Rheum Dis 2005;64:875–880.

11 Levinson JE, Wallace CA: Dismantling the pyramid. J Rheumatol 1992;19(suppl 33):6–10.

12 French AR, Mason T, Nelson AM, O'Fallon WM, Gabriel SE: Increased mortality in adults with a history of juvenile rheumatoid arthritis: a population-based study. Arthritis Rheum 2001;44:523–527.

13 Thomas E, Symmons DP, Brewster DH, Black RJ, Macfarlane GJ: National study of cause-specific mortality in rheumatoid arthritis, juvenile chronic arthritis, and other rheumatic conditions: a 20 year followup study. J Rheumatol 2003;30:958–965.

14 Minden K, Kiessling U, Listing J, Niewerth M, Döring E, Meincke J, Schöntube M, Zink A: Prognosis of patients with juvenile chronic arthritis and juvenile spondyloarthropathy. J Rheumatol 2000;27:2256–2263.

15 Oen K, Reed M, Malleson PN, Cabral DA, Petty RE, Rosenberg AM, Cheang M: Radiologic outcome and its relationship to functional disability in juvenile rheumatoid arthritis. J Rheumatol 2003;30:832–840.

16 Zak M, Hassager C, Lovell DJ, Nielsen S, Henderson CJ, Pedersen FK: Assessment of bone mineral density in adults with a history of juvenile chronic arthritis: a cross-sectional long-term followup study. Arthritis Rheum 1999;42:790–798.

17 Haugen M, Lien G, Flatø B, Kvammen J, Vinje O, Sørskaar D, Førre O: Young adults with juvenile arthritis in remission attain normal peak bone mass at the lumbar spine and forearm. Arthritis Rheum 2000;43:1504–1510.

18 Bartram S, Foster H, Francis R: Bone mineral density and juvenile chronic arthritis: comment on the article by Zak et al. Arthritis Rheum 2000;43:710.

19 French AR, Mason T, Nelson AM, Crowson CS, O'Fallon WM, Khosla S, Gabriel SE: Osteopenia in adults with a history of juvenile rheumatoid arthritis. A population based study. J Rheumatol 2002;29:1065–1070.

20 Still GF. On a form of chronic joint disease in children. Am J Dis Child 1978;132:195–200 [reprinted from Medico-Chirurgical Transactions, 1897, vol 80].

21 Simon D, Fernando C, Czernichow P, Prieur AM: Linear growth and final height in patients with systemic juvenile idiopathic arthritis treated with longterm glucocorticoids. J Rheumatol 2002;29:1296–1300.

22 Lovell DJ, White PH: Growth and nutrition in juvenile rheumatoid arthritis; in Woo P, White PH, Ansell BM (eds): Pediatric Rheumatology Update. Oxford, Oxford University Press, 1990, pp 47–56.

23 Gäre BA, Fasth A: The natural history of juvenile chronic arthritis: a population based cohort study. II. Outcome. J Rheumatol 1995; 22:308–319.

24 Zak M, Müller J, Karup Pedersen F: Final height, armspan, subischial leg length and body proportions in juvenile chronic arthritis. A long-term follow-up study. Horm Res 1999;52:80–85.

25 Saurenmann RK, Levin AV, Feldman BM, Rose JB, Laxer RM, Schneider R, Silverman ED: Prevalence, risk factors, and outcome of uveitis in juvenile idiopathic arthritis: a long-term followup study. Arthritis Rheum 2007;56:647–657.

26 Minden K: Prognosis of rheumatic diseases in children and adolescents [in German]. Kinder- und Jugendarzt 2008;8:258–266.

HORMONE RESEARCH

Horm Res 2009;72(suppl 1):26–29
DOI: 10.1159/000229760

Published online: November 27, 2009

The Impact of Chronic Inflammation on the Growing Skeleton: Lessons from Interleukin-6 Transgenic Mice

F. De Benedetti

Laboratory of Rheumatology, Direzione Scientifica, IRCCS Ospedale Pediatrico Bambino Gesù, Rome, Italy

Key Words
Inflammation · Bone · Growth · Osteoporosis · Interleukin-6

Abstract
Background: Chronic inflammatory diseases in children are associated with impairment of linear growth and bone mineral accrual. In addition to poor nutrition, reduced mobility and glucocorticoid treatment, several observations in patients suggest that inflammation itself may have a direct detrimental effect on the growing skeletal system. Among the various inflammatory cytokines produced during the inflammatory response, data in animals suggest that interleukin-6 (IL-6) may mediate the effects of inflammation on the developing skeleton. Mice overexpressing IL-6 during the prepubertal stage show stunted growth, abnormalities of the insulin-like growth factor I system, defective growth plates, delayed development of ossification centres, uncoupling of osteoblast and osteoclast activity and defective ossification. These changes appear to mirror the features observed in children with chronic inflammatory diseases. ***Conclusions:*** The tissue, cellular and molecular abnormalities reviewed provide a rationale for therapeutic approaches aimed at correcting the detrimental effects of inflammation on the developing skeletal system.

Introduction

During childhood, diseases with chronic or recurrent inflammation, such as juvenile idiopathic arthritis (JIA), inflammatory bowel diseases and cystic fibrosis, have a detrimental effect on skeletal development. This has two important long-term consequences: stunted linear growth leading to reduced adult height with a negative impact on self-esteem, particularly in adolescents, and defective bone mineral accrual, which is a risk factor for low-impact pathological fractures during childhood and also for subsequent reduction in peak bone mass and premature osteoporosis in adulthood. Many factors including prolonged immobilization, altered nutritional status, disease-related endocrine abnormalities and glucocorticoid (GC) therapy appear to be involved in the impaired skeletal development seen in children with chronic inflammatory diseases.

Moreover, several clinical observations suggest that inflammation itself negatively affects skeletal development and linear growth. In patients with JIA, linear growth is impaired during disease activity and increased during remission [1]. Response to growth hormone (GH) treatment in patients with JIA has been reported to be inversely related to the inflammatory activity of the disease as measured by the median C-reactive protein level during the treatment period [2]. Moreover, various studies in patients with JIA showed a correlation between dis-

KARGER

Fax +41 61 306 12 34
E-Mail karger@karger.ch
www.karger.com

Accessible online at:
www.karger.com/hre

Dr. Fabrizio De Benedetti
Laboratory of Rheumatology, Direzione Scientifica
IRCCS Ospedale Pediatrico Bambino Gesù, Piazza S. Onofrio 4
IT–00165 Rome (Italy)
Tel. +39 0382 502 703, Fax +39 0382 527 976, E-Mail f.debenedetti@smatteo.pv.it

ease activity and low bone mass [3]. In patients with Crohn's disease, growth impairment may occur before the onset of overt clinical features and prospective studies show that growth failure correlates strongly with disease activity, while correlation with GC intake produced conflicting results [4]. In patients with cystic fibrosis, growth impairment has been shown to correlate with the number and severity of pulmonary infections and not with the degree of pancreatic failure. Total body bone mineral deficit was correlated with disease severity and not with GC intake [5, 6].

Together, these observations suggest that factors produced during chronic inflammation affect the growing skeleton. A variety of cytokines released during the inflammatory response are potential candidates. Interleukin (IL)-1, IL-6 and tumor necrosis factor (TNF) have been shown to affect signaling in chondrocytes [7]. These cytokines, as well as others, may affect the coupling of osteoclast and osteoblast activities [8]. Several lines of evidence point to a major role of IL-6 in the systemic effects of chronic inflammation on the growing skeleton. We will briefly review the biology of IL-6 as a systemically active cytokine and present the evidence in animal models suggesting a major role of IL-6 in mediating the effects of chronic inflammation on the maturing skeleton.

IL-6 as a Systemically Active Cytokine

The major role of IL-6 in mediating the systemic features of chronic inflammation depends on the mode of functioning of the IL-6 receptor system, which is rather unique in cytokine biology. First, IL-6 binds to the membrane IL-6 receptor (mIL-6R). The mIL-6R has a very short cytoplasmic tail that is unable to transduce signals. Neither IL-6 alone nor mIL-6R alone can bind to gp130, the signaling receptor subunit; however, the IL-6/IL-6R complex binds to gp130 with high affinity to form a receptor complex, which leads to gp130 dimerization and triggering of signal transduction. An alternative mechanism involves the soluble form of the IL-6R (sIL-6R). The interaction of IL-6 with sIL-6R leads to the formation of an IL-6/sIL-6R complex that binds and activates the signal-transducing subunit gp130 in a manner similar to that of the full-membrane IL-6R. Therefore, in contrast to most soluble cytokine receptors, sIL-6R behaves as an agonist (or as a cocytokine), and a vast body of in vitro and in vivo evidence indicates that sIL-6R potentiates the effects of IL-6. The sIL-6R is present at ng/ml levels in biological fluids at steady-state physiological conditions. It is produced not only by shedding through cleavage of the full mIL-6R by inflammatory proteases, but also by differential mRNA splicing [9]. This implies the presence of a physiological mechanism independent of proteolytic cleavage by inflammatory proteins, which maintain high levels of sIL-6R. The sIL-6R captures IL-6 at sites of inflammation, functioning as a carrier protein to deliver IL-6 to organs far from the inflammatory sites. Indeed, overexpression of the sIL-6R in mice increased plasma IL-6 half-life and led to potentiation and prolongation of IL-6 activities.

Overexpression of IL-6 in Mice Causes Stunted Growth and Decreased Insulin-Like Growth Factor I

Four different strains of IL-6 transgenic mice have shown stunted growth. One of these strains, the NSE/hIL6 transgenic mouse, has been characterized in great detail [10]. Beginning at birth, these mice express elevated levels of circulating human IL-6 that are constant regardless of inflammatory stimuli. Other inflammatory cytokines, such as IL-1 or TNF, are undetectable. These mice have severely stunted linear growth with an adult size that is 30–50% smaller as compared with nontransgenic littermates [10]. This defect is completely reversed by antagonizing IL-6, proving that it is IL-6 dependent [11]. Food intake and glucose levels are normal. Similar to observations in children with JIA or other chronic inflammatory diseases, these mice have normal GH production, but low plasma levels of insulin-like growth factor I (IGF-I). The effect of IL-6 on circulating IGF-I levels is not due to reduced hepatic IGF-I production, but rather to an accelerated peripheral clearance due to increased proteolysis of IGF-binding protein 3 (IGFBP-3) [12]. In patients with systemic JIA, childhood Crohn's disease and perinatal human immunodeficiency virus infection, an inverse correlation has been found between circulating IL-6 and both IGF-I and IGFBP-3 levels – suggesting that the mechanism described in this mouse model may indeed reproduce the effect of IL-6 on the GH/IGF-I axis in vivo during chronic inflammation [12].

The role of IL-6 in causing stunted growth has also been demonstrated in a rat model of inflammatory colitis. Prepubertal rats showed impaired linear growth following the induction of experimental colitis [13]. The defective growth was at least partially reversed by administration of a neutralizing antibody to IL-6. These results imply that, in the context of chronic tissue inflammation, IL-6 plays a major role in causing stunted growth.

In the rat model, circulating IGF-I levels were decreased [13]. However, in contrast with the IL-6 transgenic mice, liver IGF-I protein expression in rats was reduced. TNF has been shown to decrease in vivo liver IGF-I expression [14]. Therefore, it is conceivable that, within the context of inflammation, various inflammatory cytokines have an impact on IGF-I availability.

Overexpression of IL-6 in Mice Causes Abnormalities in the Growth Plate and in Endochondral Ossification

Although the relevance of circulating versus locally produced IGF-I remains to be established, IGF-I is a mediator involved in cartilage growth. In IL-6 transgenic mice, the growth plates were thinner, with a markedly reduced hypertrophic zone [15]. Since the growth plate has a major role in longitudinal bone growth, this finding could contribute to stunted growth. The growth plate defect may be mediated by an abnormal IGF-I level or may be secondary to a direct effect of IL-6 on the growth plate. While IL-6 has been shown to affect matrix protein production by articular chondrocytes, no data regarding the effect of IL-6 on growth plate chondrocytes are available. IL-6 transgenic mice also showed delayed formation of epiphyseal ossification centres with defective mineralization, delayed appearance of blood vessels and delayed colonization by bone marrow cells [15]. We hypothesize that the defective formation of epiphyseal ossification centres in IL-6 transgenic mice mirrors the well-known delayed skeletal age observed in patients with chronic inflammatory diseases.

Overexpression of IL-6 in Mice Causes Uncoupling of Osteoclast and Osteoblast Activity and Decreased Trabecular and Cortical Bone Formation

In the IL-6 transgenic mice, histochemistry showed an increased number of osteoclasts and mononuclear osteoclast precursors lining bone trabeculae. Increased bone marrow osteoclastogenesis was also observed. Elevated levels of urinary deoxypyridinoline (DPD) indicated increased bone resorption [15]. These observations in IL-6 transgenic mice are consistent with a vast body of evidence demonstrating a major role of IL-6 in inducing and activating osteoclasts. In vitro, IL-6 induces functionally active (i.e., pit-forming) osteoclasts from mononuclear cells [16] and increases bone resorption in whole-organ cultures of calvaria bone [17]. IL-6 knockout (IL-6–/–) mice are protected from ovariectomy-induced bone loss, and this protection is associated with a marked reduction in osteoclasts [18]. Incidentally, IL-6–/– mice do not have an overt bone phenotype [19], suggesting that, at steady-state physiological conditions, IL-6 does not appear to play a major role in bone homeostasis. In IL-6 transgenic mice, osteoblasts were smaller and fewer, and low serum osteocalcin levels indicated decreased bone deposition. In vitro, IL-6 inhibits the function of osteoblasts through formation of mineralized nodules, but it does not appear to inhibit differentiation or proliferation [15].

The imbalance between osteoclast and osteoblast activity in IL-6 transgenic mice leads to significant osteopenia with reduced trabecular and cortical bone formation [15]. In these mice, the balance between resorption and deposition is physiologically skewed in favor of resorption rather than deposition (which would allow growth). Evaluation of the mineral apposition rate showed a marked defect in ossification. Moreover, serum osteocalcin levels correlated directly with body weight while urinary DPD levels correlated inversely with body weight [15]. This indicates that the imbalance in bone cell activities appears to limit bone growth and, therefore, has a tangible effect on linear growth.

Conclusions

Transgenic mice with high levels of circulating IL-6 during the prepubertal stage show stunted growth, abnormalities of the IGF-I system, defective growth plates, delayed development of ossification centres, uncoupling of osteoblasts and osteoclast activity and defective ossification. These observations suggest that, at least in animals, selective overexpression of IL-6 in the absence of chronic inflammation and other inflammatory cytokines causes abnormalities of the growing skeleton similar to those observed in children with chronic inflammatory diseases. Although other proinflammatory cytokines, such as IL-1 and TNF, are also overproduced in chronic inflammatory diseases, to date there have been no studies in animal models showing a direct link between chronic production of these two cytokines and stunted growth or defective ossification.

Furthermore, clinical observations in patients support a direct link between IL-6 and the effect of chronic inflammation on the developing skeleton. In patients with cystic fibrosis, IL-6 levels have been found to be associated with decreased bone mineral content gain and increased bone resorption as indicated by DPD levels [20, 21]. In a prospective study, we found that mean IL-6 levels inversely correlated with osteoblast activity as measured by bone alkaline phosphatase activity [F. De Benedetti, unpublished data, 2008]. IL-6 is the factor responsible for the ability of sera from patients with Crohn's disease to inhibit bone mineralization in vitro [22]. Moreover, in these patients, a high-producing IL-6 promoter polymorphism (associated with increased IL-6 production) correlated inversely with stature [13].

In conclusion, together with observations in patients with chronic inflammatory diseases, data in animal models suggest that elevated production of IL-6 appears to be a generalized mechanism by which inflammation affects the developing skeleton. Therapies aimed at correcting the detrimental effects on the developing skeleton should focus on better control of the inflammatory activity of the underlying disease or interference with the cellular and molecular abnormalities induced by IL-6.

Disclosure Statement

The author declares membership on advisory committees or review panels and honoraria received from Roche.

References

1 Ansell BM, Bywaters EG: Growth in Still's disease. Ann Rheum Dis 1956;15:295–319.
2 Davies UM, Rooney M, Preece MA, Ansell BM, Woo P: Treatment of growth retardation in juvenile chronic arthritis with recombinant human growth hormone. J Rheumatol 1994;21:153–158.
3 Burnham JM, Shults J, Dubner SE, Sembhi H, Zemel BS, Leonard MB: Bone density, structure, and strength in juvenile idiopathic arthritis: importance of disease severity and muscle deficits. Arthritis Rheum 2008;58:2518–2527.
4 Cezard JP, Touati G, Alberti C, Hugot JP, Brinon C, Czernichow P: Growth in paediatric Crohn's disease. Horm Res 2002;58(suppl 1):11–15.
5 Henderson RC, Madsen CD: Bone mineral content and body composition in children and young adults with cystic fibrosis. Pediatr Pulmonol 1999;27:80–84.
6 Sproul A, Huang N: Growth patterns in children with cystic fibrosis. J Pediatr 1964;65:664–676.
7 MacRae VE, Farquharson C, Ahmed SF: The pathophysiology of the growth plate in juvenile idiopathic arthritis. Rheumatology (Oxford) 2006;45:11–19.
8 Walsh MC, Kim N, Kadono Y, Rho J, Lee SY, Lorenzo J, Choi Y: Osteoimmunology: interplay between the immune system and bone metabolism. Annu Rev Immunol 2006;24:33–63.
9 Rose-John S, Scheller J, Elson G, Jones SA: Interleukin-6 biology is coordinated by membrane-bound and soluble receptors: role in inflammation and cancer. J Leuk Biol 2006;80:227–236.
10 De Benedetti F, Alonzi T, Moretta A, Lazzaro D, Costa P, Poli V, Martini A, Ciliberto G, Fattori E: Interleukin 6 causes growth impairment in transgenic mice through a decrease in insulin-like growth factor-I. A model for stunted growth in children with chronic inflammation. J Clin Invest 1997;99:643–650.
11 De Benedetti F, Pignatti P, Vivarelli M, Meazza C, Ciliberto G, Savino R, Martini A: In vivo neutralization of human IL-6 (hIL-6) achieved by immunization of hIL-6-transgenic mice with a hIL-6 receptor antagonist. J Immunol 2001;166:4334–4340.
12 De Benedetti F, Meazza C, Oliveri M, Pignatti P, Vivarelli M, Alonzi T, Fattori E, Garrone S, Barreca A, Martini A: Effect of IL-6 on IGF binding protein-3: a study in IL-6 transgenic mice and in patients with systemic juvenile idiopathic arthritis. Endocrinology 2001;142:4818–4826.
13 Sawczenko A, Azooz O, Paraszczuk J, Idestrom M, Croft NM, Savage MO, Ballinger AB, Sanderson IR: Intestinal inflammation-induced growth retardation acts through IL-6 in rats and depends on the -174 IL-6 G/C polymorphism in children. Proc Natl Acad Sci USA 2005;102:13260–13265.
14 Yumet G, Shumate ML, Bryant P, Lin CM, Lang CH, Cooney RN: Tumor necrosis factor mediates hepatic growth hormone resistance during sepsis. Am J Physiol 2002;283:E472–E481.
15 De Benedetti F, Rucci N, Del Fattore A, Peruzzi B, Paro R, Longo M, Vivarelli M, Muratori F, Berni S, Ballanti P, Ferrari S, Teti A: Impaired skeletal development in interleukin-6-transgenic mice: a model for the impact of chronic inflammation on the growing skeletal system. Arthritis Rheum 2006;54:3551–3563.
16 Tamura T, Udagawa N, Takahashi N, Miyaura C, Tanaka S, Yamada Y, Koishihara Y, Ohsugi Y, Kumaki K, Taga T, Kishimoto T, Suda T: Soluble interleukin-6 receptor triggers osteoclast formation by interleukin 6. Proc Natl Acad Sci USA 1993;90:11924–11928.
17 Palmqvist P, Persson E, Conaway HH, Lerner UH: IL-6, leukemia inhibitory factor, and oncostatin M stimulate bone resorption and regulate the expression of receptor activator of NF-kappa B ligand, osteoprotegerin, and receptor activator of NF-kappa B in mouse calvariae. J Immunol 2002;169:3353–3362.
18 Poli V, Balena R, Fattori E, Markatos A, Yamamoto M, Tanaka H, Ciliberto G, Rodan GA, Costantini F: Interleukin-6 deficient mice are protected from bone loss caused by estrogen depletion. EMBO J 1994;13:1189–1196.
19 Dai J, Lin D, Zhang J, Habib P, Smith P, Murtha J, Fu Z, Yao Z, Qi Y, Keller ET: Chronic alcohol ingestion induces osteoclastogenesis and bone loss through IL-6 in mice. J Clin Invest 2000;106:887–895.
20 Aris RM, Stephens AR, Ontjes DA, Denene Blackwood A, Lark RK, Hensler MB, Neuringer IP, Lester GE: Adverse alterations in bone metabolism are associated with lung infection in adults with cystic fibrosis. Am J Respir Crit Care Med 2000;162:1674–1678.
21 Haworth CS, Selby PL, Webb AK, Martin L, Elborn JS, Sharples LD, Adams JE: Inflammatory related changes in bone mineral content in adults with cystic fibrosis. Thorax 2004;59:613–617.
22 Sylvester FA, Wyzga N, Hyams JS, Gronowicz GA: Effect of Crohn's disease on bone metabolism in vitro: a role for interleukin-6. J Bone Miner Res 2002;17:695–702.

HORMONE RESEARCH

Horm Res 2009;72(suppl 1):30–35
DOI: 10.1159/000229761

Published online: November 27, 2009

Mechanisms of Impaired Growth: Effect of Steroids on Bone and Cartilage

Robert C. Olney

Division of Pediatric Endocrinology, Nemours Children's Clinic, Jacksonville, Fla., USA

Key Words
Glucocorticoids · Osteoblasts · Osteoclasts · Chondrocytes · Growth

Abstract
Background: Long-term treatment with high-dose glucocorticoids (GCs) has profound effects on bone metabolism and linear growth. Bone metabolism is a balance between bone resorption by osteoclasts and new bone formation by osteoblasts. Systemically, GC treatment reduces circulating levels of estrogen and modestly increases parathyroid hormone levels. At the local level, GCs decrease insulin-like growth factor I (IGF-I) production, induce IGF-I resistance and increase nuclear factor κB ligand production by osteoblasts. These alterations inhibit new bone formation and stimulate bone resorption, with a net loss of bone over time. Clinically, this results in decreased bone mineral density, osteoporosis and increased risk for fracture. Local effects of GCs at the growth plate include reduction of IGF-I production, inducing IGF-I resistance and reducing production of C-type natriuretic peptide, which results in a reduction of chondrocyte proliferation, matrix synthesis and hypertrophy. These reductions in chondrocyte function result in decreased linear growth. ***Conclusions:*** The effects of GCs on bone metabolism and linear growth are sensitive and specific and represent an evolutionary adaptation to redirect resources during times of physiologic stress. Since many of these effects result from alterations in IGF-I production, growth hormone therapy is a potential approach to ameliorate these problems.

Introduction

Long-term treatment with high-dose glucocorticoids (GCs) is bad for bones. Such treatment results in reduced bone mineral density, osteoporosis and increased risk for fractures, as well as linear growth failure in children. Yet, the treatment of chronic inflammatory diseases (such as juvenile idiopathic arthritis) often requires the potent anti-inflammatory effects of these drugs. This report briefly reviews the effects of high-dose GCs on bone and cartilage in children and provides a background for understanding how growth hormone therapy might ameliorate some of these effects.

Effect of GCs on Bone Metabolism

Bone maintenance is the continuous processes of bone resorption by osteoclasts and new bone formation by osteoblasts. GCs alter the balance between these processes, resulting in a net loss of bone. The regulatory processes of bone maintenance and the effect of GCs are complex; therefore, a complete discussion is beyond the scope of this report. Several recent reviews cover these topics in greater detail [1–3], while this article focuses primarily on the regulatory systems affected by GCs.

Bone Formation: Osteoblast Function and Regulation

Osteoblasts go through a life cycle of recruitment from precursors, proliferation and anabolic function and either apoptosis or further differentiation into osteocytes

KARGER

Fax +41 61 306 12 34
E-Mail karger@karger.ch
www.karger.com

0301–0163/09/0727–0030$26.00/0

Accessible online at:
www.karger.com/hre

Robert C. Olney
Division of Pediatric Endocrinology
Nemours Children's Clinic, 807 Children's Way
Jacksonville, FL 32207 (USA)
Tel. +1 904 390 3600, Fax +1 904 390 3699, E-Mail rolney@nemours.org

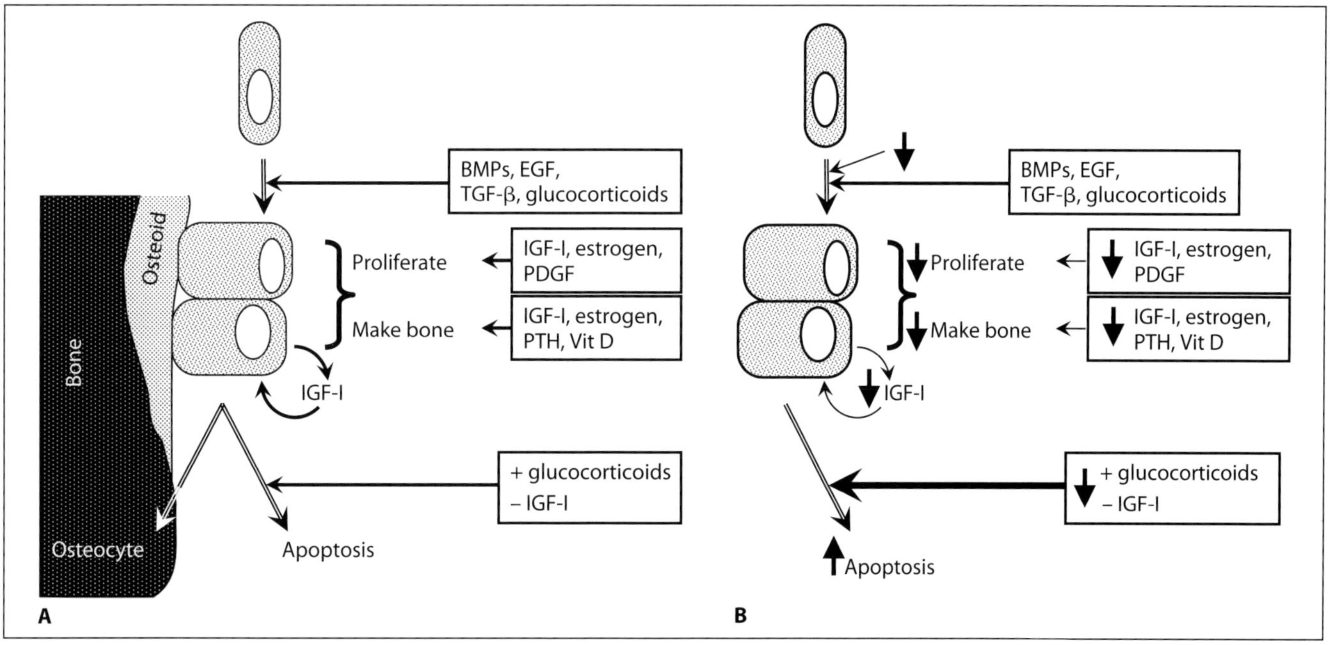

Fig. 1. Bone formation: osteoblasts. **A** Regulation of osteoblasts. Osteoblasts are recruited from mesenchymal stem cell precursors under the stimulation of BMPs, EGF, TGF-β and GCs. Young osteoblasts undergo proliferation in response to IGF-I, estrogen and PDGF. The anabolic actions of laying down osteoid matrix and directing mineralization are regulated by IGF-I, estrogen, PTH and vitamin D. IGF-I is also produced by osteoblasts, acting in both an endocrine and paracrine manner to stimulate proliferation and anabolic function. Osteoblasts are then either caught up in the newly formed bone and differentiate further to osteocytes or undergo apoptosis. GCs stimulate and IGF-I inhibits apoptosis. **B** Effect of GCs on osteoblasts. Systemically, GCs reduce estrogen levels. GCs have a direct effect of reducing locally produced IGF-I and inducing IGF-I resistance, reducing osteoblast proliferation and anabolic function. The reduction of IGF-I effect increases osteoblast apoptosis. The net result is a reduction in the number of osteoblasts and of anabolic function, reducing new bone formation. BMP = Bone morphogenetic protein; EGF = epithelial growth factor; TGF-β = transforming growth factor β; IGF-I = insulin-like growth factor I; PDGF = platelet-derived growth factor; PTH = parathyroid hormone.

(fig. 1) [4]. Osteoblasts are derived from mesenchymal (stromal) stem cells found primarily in bone marrow. Following differentiation, osteoblasts still have the capacity to proliferate. Differentiated osteoblasts line bone surfaces and secrete osteoid matrix, which is rich in collagen and proteoglycans. This matrix serves as the scaffolding for mineralization and true bone formation. Osteoblasts also produce the machinery necessary for mineralization, including alkaline phosphatase and osteocalcin. Interestingly, the actual process of mineralization does not occur directly adjacent to the osteoblast, but a short distance away. This process results in a thin layer of new bone being added to existing bone.

Osteoblasts also direct bone resorption by secreting receptor activator of nuclear factor κB ligand (RANKL), an activator of osteoclasts, and osteoprotegerin (OPG), a competitive inhibitor of RANKL. Osteoblasts have two potential fates. A small fraction are caught up in the newly formed bone and differentiate further into osteocytes, which primarily serve a mechanosensing and communication function within bone. The majority of osteoblasts, however, undergo apoptosis.

Osteoblasts are regulated by multiple systemic and local factors [4]. The differentiation of stem cells into osteoblasts is regulated by bone morphogenetic proteins (BMPs), epithelial growth factor (EGF), transforming growth factor-β (TGF-β) and GCs. Proliferation of osteoblasts is regulated by such factors as insulin-like growth factor I (IGF-I), platelet-derived growth factor (PDGF) and estrogen. The anabolic functions of osteoblasts are also regulated by IGF-I and estrogen, as well as parathyroid hormone (PTH) and vitamin D. Osteoblasts produce IGF-I, which works through both endocrine and paracrine mechanisms. Apoptosis is regulated, in part, through GCs and IGF-I.

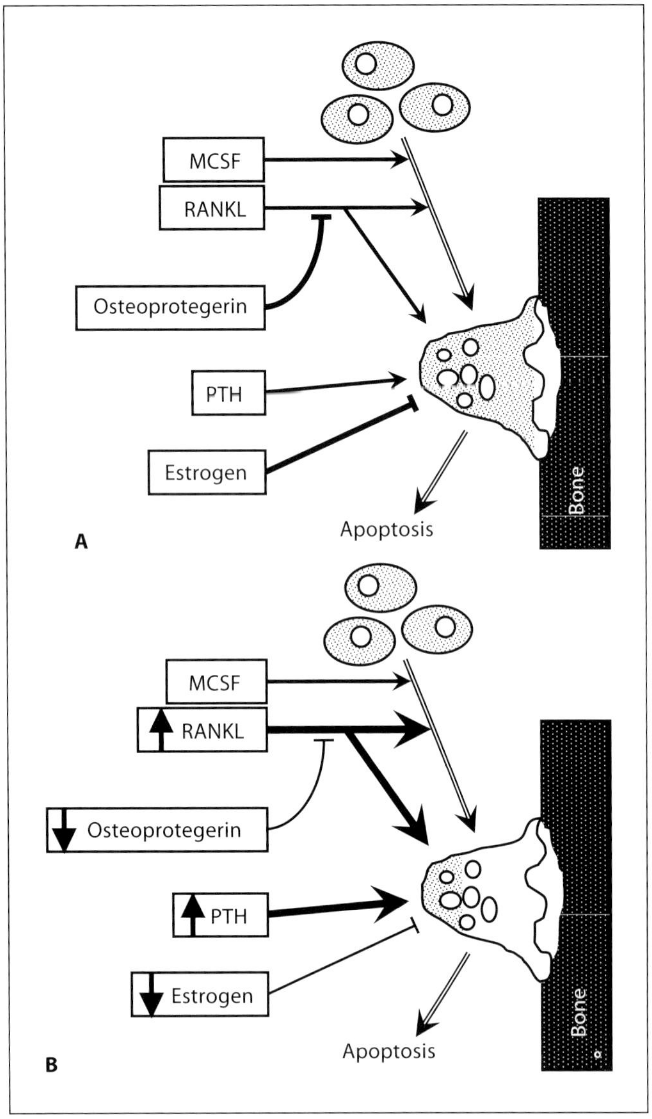

Fig. 2. Bone resorption: osteoclasts. **A** Regulation of osteoclasts. Osteoclasts are recruited from macrophage precursors under the stimulation of MCSF and RANKL and coalesce into multinucleated giant cells. RANKL and its inhibitor, OPG, derive in part from osteoblasts. RANKL production is regulated by estrogen. Bone resorption actions are stimulated by RANKL and PTH and are directly inhibited by estrogen. At the end of their life cycle, osteoclasts undergo apoptosis. **B** Effect of GCs on osteoclasts. The systemic reduction of estrogen by GCs results in increased RANKL production by osteoblasts and a loss of estrogen inhibition of osteoclast activity. Decreased OPG also decreases this inhibition. GCs cause a modest increase in PTH levels, further increasing osteoclast activity. The net result is an increased number of osteoclasts and increased osteoclast activity, resulting in increased bone resorption. MCSF = Macrophage colony-stimulating factor; RANKL = receptor activator of nuclear factor κB ligand; PTH = parathyroid hormone.

Effect of GCs on Osteoblasts

Each of the steps in the osteoblast life cycle is affected by high-dose GCs (fig. 1B) [1, 2]. GCs directly inhibit stem cell differentiation into osteoblasts. Systemically, GCs induce resistance to IGF-I, as demonstrated by increased serum IGF-I levels [5, 6]. They also inhibit pituitary gonadotropin production, causing relative hypogonadism [7]. Further, GCs decrease osteoblast production of local IGF-I [8]. The resulting decreases in IGF-I, IGF-I effect and estrogen result in decreased osteoblast proliferation and anabolic functions. Finally, the combination of GCs with reduced IGF-I effect stimulates osteoblast apoptosis. The net result is that there are fewer osteoblasts present and remaining osteoblasts have decreased anabolic activity, resulting in a decrease in new bone formation. Conversely, GCs directly affect osteoblasts by increasing RANKL and decreasing OPG production, leading to increased stimulation of osteoclasts and bone resorption.

Bone Resorption: Osteoclast Function and Regulation

Osteoclasts are part of the monocytic/macrophage family and derive primarily from bone marrow macrophages (fig. 2) [9]. During differentiation, the cells coalesce into multinucleated giant cells. The mature osteoclast attaches itself to a bone surface, creating a microenvironment between cell and bone. Protons are pumped into this space, creating a highly acidic environment. The acid leaches minerals from the matrix and specific enzymes (i.e., cathepsin K, matrix metalloproteases, tartrate-resistant acid phosphatase, etc.) digest the matrix itself. During this process, the osteoclast burrows down, resorbing bone as it goes. The osteoclast completes its life cycle by undergoing apoptosis.

Osteoblasts and osteoclasts work in close proximity to one another, creating a 'bone-forming unit'. In this functional unit, a number of osteoclasts work together to form a tunnel within existing bone. Osteoblasts follow behind, lining the tunnel walls and laying down new bone. Through the action of thousands of these bone-forming units, bone is continually remodeled [9].

As with osteoblasts, osteoclast regulation is also complex [9]. Macrophage colony-stimulating factor (MCSF) and RANKL are required for precursor recruitment and are produced by osteoblasts and their mesenchymal precursors. RANKL, PTH and GCs stimulate the bone resorption functions of the osteoclast. These functions are inhibited by OPG, which is also produced by osteoblasts. Estrogen has a direct inhibitory effect on osteoclasts, and it also acts on osteoblasts to decrease RANKL production.

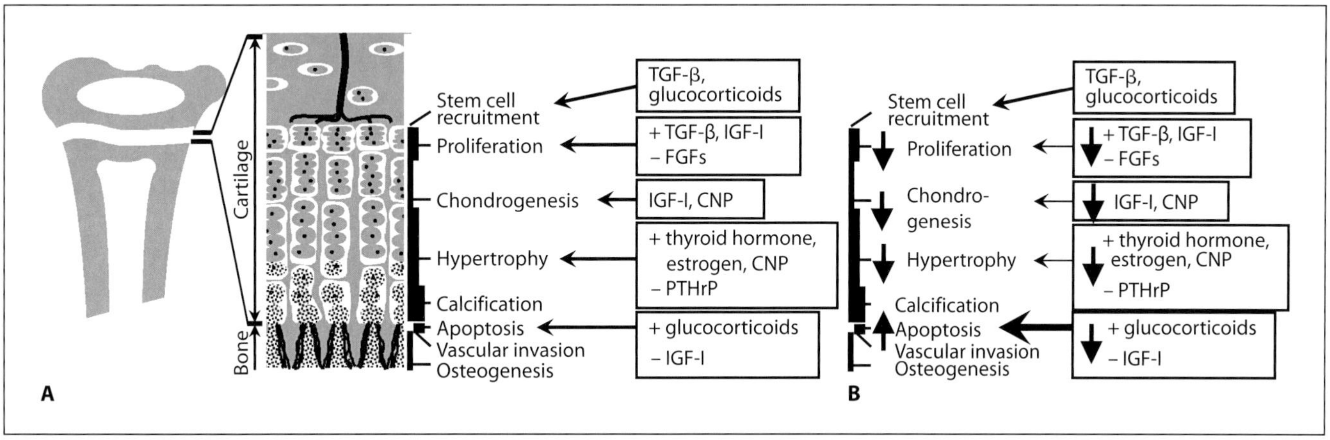

Fig. 3. Linear growth: the growth plate. **A** Regulation of the growth plate. Chondrogenic stem cells are recruited into the columnar zone of the growth plate under the stimulation of TGF-β, IHH and GCs. The young chondrocytes undergo a phase of proliferation in an oriented manner, establishing the columns within the growth plate. Proliferation is stimulated by TGF-β and IGF-I and inhibited by FGFs. In the columnar zone, chondrocytes produce cartilage matrix consisting of collagens and proteoglycans under the regulation of IGF-I and CNP. Chondrocytes undergo further differentiation ('hypertrophy') in a process stimulated by thyroid hormone, estrogen, and CNP and inhibited by PTHrP. IGF-I, CNP and PTHrP are produced locally in the growth plate, working in a paracrine manner. Hypertrophic chondrocytes produce an altered cartilage matrix that allows for provisional calcification and vascular invasion. The chondrocytes then undergo apoptosis stimulated by GCs and inhibited by IGF-I. Osteoblasts are recruited to remodel the calcified cartilage matrix into true bone. **B** Effect of GCs on the growth plate. The systemic reduction in estrogen (in adolescents) slows chondrocyte hypertrophy. Locally, GCs reduce local IGF-I production and induce IGF-I resistance. Local production of CNP production is also reduced. The result is decreased chondrocyte proliferation, matrix synthesis and hypertrophy, resulting in slowed linear growth. TGF-β = Transforming growth factor-β; IHH = Indian hedgehog (signaling); GC = glucocorticoid; IGF-I = insulin-like growth factor-I; FGF = fibroblast growth factor; CNP = C-type natriuretic peptide; PTHrP = parathyroid hormone-related peptide.

Effect of GCs on Osteoclasts

Through reduction of estrogen and by direct effects of GCs on osteoblasts, RANKL production is increased and OPG production is decreased (fig. 2B). This results in increased precursor recruitment and increased osteoclast activity. Further, GCs induce a mild decrease in calcium uptake in the kidney, causing a slight increase in PTH levels [10]. This increase in PTH also increases osteoclast activity. Hence, the net result is an increase in the number of osteoclasts, each with increased catabolic activity.

Net Effect of GCs on Bone

The effect of steroids on bone is the result of imbalance between bone formation and resorption. GCs reduce recruitment of osteoblasts from precursors, reduce osteoblast proliferation, reduce the anabolic activity of osteoblasts and increase osteoblast apoptosis. These drugs also increase osteoclast recruitment from precursors and increase osteoclast catabolic activity. The resulting decrease in bone formation and increase in bone resorption eventually result in loss of bone mineral density, development of osteoporosis and increased risk for fracture.

Effect of GCs on Growth

High-dose GCs cause profound linear growth failure. Linear growth is the result of a complex series of events that occurs within the epiphyseal growth plates, located at the ends of the long bones. Similar to the effects of GCs on bone metabolism, the effects of GCs on the growth plate are complex. Interested readers are referred to in-depth reviews by van der Eerden et al. and Hochberg [11, 12].

Growth: Growth Plate Function and Regulation

The growth plate can be divided into several histologically different zones and the chondrocytes found within each zone have different characteristics (fig. 3). The chondrocytes of the reserve zone are not very active metabolically and do not divide rapidly. Chondrogenic stem cells lie at the junction of the reserve zone and proliferative zone. These stem cells likely derive from mesenchymal stem cells. Although the true source is unclear, many researchers believe that these stem cells arise from cells within the reserve zone. The stem cells divide in a uniform plane, giving rise to the daughter cell columns in the proliferative zone. Here, chondrocytes undergo rapid division and cartilage matrix production. The proliferative phase is followed by a phase of transition, known variously as 'postmitotic', 'prehypertrophic' or 'transitional' chondrocytes. Further maturation results in chondrocyte hypertrophy. Chondrocytes in the hypertrophic zone show increased production of collagen type X, alkaline phosphatase and matrix metalloproteases and give rise to matrix vesicles, which initiate matrix calcification. By producing these substances, the hypertrophic chondrocytes alter the structure of the surrounding cartilage matrix and begin the process of calcification. The altered matrix then allows for vascularization. Osteoblasts subsequently infiltrate and complete the ossification process, while the hypertrophic chondrocytes undergo apoptosis. The sum of the results of the proliferative and hypertrophic phases of growth plate chondrocytes is bone growth [11].

Recruitment of mesenchymal stem cells into chondrocytes is mediated by TGF-β, Indian hedgehog signaling and GCs. Subsequent proliferation is mediated by TGF-β, IGF-I and PDGF and inhibited by fibroblast growth factors. Cartilage matrix synthesis is most potently regulated by IGF-I. In rodents, IGF-I is also produced in the growth plate and, as in the case of osteoblasts, works in both an endocrine and paracrine manner. However, in bovine [13] and human [R.C. Olney, unpublished data, 2001] growth plate chondrocytes, IGF-I expression cannot be demonstrated. Whether IGF-I is produced in the human growth plate remains somewhat controversial.

The transition into hypertrophic chondrocytes is regulated systemically by thyroid hormone and estrogen. Studies in recent years have shown that this transition is also regulated by local feedback loops. Indian hedgehog is expressed and secreted by hypertrophic chondrocytes. It then diffuses up the growth plate to the late proliferative and prehypertrophic zones and (prenatally) to the perichondrium, where signaling increases the expression and secretion of PTH-related peptide. This peptide then acts on prehypertrophic chondrocytes to inhibit hypertrophic differentiation, completing the feedback loop [14]. Details of an opposing feedback loop are emerging, where C-type natriuretic peptide (CNP) is produced in hypertrophic chondrocytes and possibly metaphyseal osteoblasts, and it then diffuses up the growth plate to bind to natriuretic peptide receptor-B on chondrocytes in the proliferative zone [15]. This signaling stimulates matrix synthesis and differentiation of chondrocytes into hypertrophy. Apoptosis of the hypertrophic chondrocyte is inhibited by IGF-I and stimulated by GCs.

Effect of GCs on the Growth Plate

The effect of high-dose GCs on stem cell recruitment is unknown. GCs inhibit Akt-phosphatidylinositol 3-kinase pathway signaling, resulting in decreased differentiation of chondrocyte precursors [16] and increasing apoptosis in mature chondrocytes [17] in vitro. Since IGF-I signals, in part, through this pathway, this may represent the mechanism of IGF-I resistance in these cells [17]. GCs induce a rapid decrease in CNP production [18], although whether or not this is a direct effect is unknown. Reduced IGF-I effect and CNP levels reduce cartilage matrix production. The systemic reduction of estrogen and the local reduction of CNP reduce chondrocyte differentiation into the hypertrophic zone. Chondrocyte apoptosis is increased with GCs and reduced IGF-I effect.

Net Effect of GCs on Growth

The net effect of GCs on the growth plate is a decrease in overall function. GCs reduce chondrocyte proliferation, cartilage matrix synthesis and hypertrophic differentiation, while increasing apoptosis. This decrease in growth plate function results in a marked reduction in linear growth.

Conclusions

High-dose GCs are bad for bones and bad for growth. The endogenous role of GCs is to prepare and support the body during times of physiologic stress. During such times, inflammation becomes a draw on resources (energy and substrate) that might be needed elsewhere, hence the anti-inflammatory effects of cortisol. Similarly, linear growth and bone formation are also draws on these resources and thus are also suppressed by this hormone. The skeleton, besides providing structural support, is also a reservoir of minerals. During times of stress, this reservoir is drawn upon by increasing bone resorption, e.g., making calcium available for optimal muscle function. From this viewpoint, the bone loss and growth-inhibiting properties of GCs are integral parts of their physiological function. It is only when anti-inflammatory GCs are given at high doses for long periods that these effects on bone and growth become 'side effects'. Many of the effects of GCs on bone and growth occur through suppression of anabolic regulatory pathways. Since the growth hormone/IGF-I system is part of these anabolic pathways, it is reasonable to explore growth hormone therapy as an approach to ameliorate these effects.

Disclosure Statement

The author has received honoraria and served as a speaker, teacher, advisory committee or review panel member for Pfizer, Eli Lilly and Genentech.

References

1 De Nijs RN: Glucocorticoid-induced osteoporosis: a review on pathophysiology and treatment options. Minerva Med 2008;99:23–43.

2 Canalis E, Mazziotti G, Giustina A, Bilezikian JP: Glucocorticoid-induced osteoporosis: pathophysiology and therapy. Osteoporos Int 2007;18:1319–1328.

3 Leonard MB: Glucocorticoid-induced osteoporosis in children: impact of the underlying disease. Pediatrics 2007;119(suppl 2):S166–S174.

4 Aubin JE, Lian JB, Stein GS: Bone formation: maturation and functional activities of osteoblast lineage cells; in Favus MJ, Lian JB, Goldring SR (eds): Primer on the Metabolic Diseases and Disorders of Mineral Metabolism. Washington DC, American Society for Bone and Mineral Research, 2006, pp 20–29.

5 Prummel MF, Wiersinga WM, Oosting H, Endert E: The effect of long-term prednisone treatment on growth hormone and insulin-like growth factor-1. J Endocrinol Invest 1996;19:620–623.

6 Wajchenberg BL, Liberman B, Giannella Neto D, Morozimato MY, Semer M, Bracco LO, Salgado LR, Knoepfelmacher M, Borges MH, Pinto AC, Kater CE, Lengyel AM: Growth hormone axis in Cushing's syndrome. Horm Res 1996;45:99–107.

7 Gore AC, Attardi B, DeFranco DB: Glucocorticoid repression of the reproductive axis: effects on GnRH and gonadotropin subunit mRNA levels. Mol Cell Endocrinol 2006;256:40–48.

8 Delany AM, Durant D, Canalis E: Glucocorticoid suppression of IGF I transcription in osteoblasts. Mol Endocrinol 2001;15:1781–1789.

9 Ross FP: Osteoclast biology and bone resorption; in Favus MJ, Lian JB, Goldring SR (eds): Primer on the Metabolic Diseases and Disorders of Mineral Metabolism. Washington DC, American Society for Bone and Mineral Research, 2006, pp 30–35.

10 Kuroki Y, Kaji H, Kawano S, Kanda F, Takai Y, Kajikawa M, Sugimoto T: Short-term effects of glucocorticoid therapy on biochemical markers of bone metabolism in Japanese patients: a prospective study. J Bone Miner Metab 2008;26:271–278.

11 van der Eerden BC, Karperien M, Wit JM: Systemic and local regulation of the growth plate. Endocr Rev 2003;24:782–801.

12 Hochberg Z: Mechanisms of steroid impairment of growth. Horm Res 2002;58(suppl 1):33–38.

13 Hutchison MR, Bassett MH, White PC: Insulin-like growth factor-I and fibroblast growth factor, but not growth hormone, affect growth plate chondrocyte proliferation. Endocrinology 2007;148:3122–3130.

14 Kronenberg HM: PTHrP and skeletal development. Ann N Y Acad Sci 2006;1068:1–13.

15 Olney RC: C-type natriuretic peptide in growth: a new paradigm. Growth Horm IGF Res 2006;16(suppl A):S6–S14.

16 Fujita T, Fukuyama R, Enomoto H, Komori T: Dexamethasone inhibits insulin-induced chondrogenesis of ATDC5 cells by preventing PI3K-Akt signaling and DNA binding of Runx2. J Cell Biochem 2004;93:374–383.

17 Chrysis D, Zaman F, Chagin AS, Takigawa M, Sävendahl L: Dexamethasone induces apoptosis in proliferative chondrocytes through activation of caspases and suppression of the Akt-phosphatidylinositol 3′-kinase signaling pathway. Endocrinology 2005;146:1391–1397.

18 Prickett TC, Lynn AM, Barrell GK, Darlow BA, Cameron VA, Espiner EA, Richards AM, Yandle TG: Amino-terminal proCNP: a putative marker of cartilage activity in postnatal growth. Pediatr Res 2005;58:334–340.

HORMONE RESEARCH

Horm Res 2009;72(suppl 1):36–41
DOI: 10.1159/000229762

Published online: November 27, 2009

Mechanisms of Muscle Atrophy Induced by Glucocorticoids

O. Schakman H. Gilson S. Kalista J.P. Thissen

Unité de Diabétologie et Nutrition, Faculté de Médecine, Université Catholique de Louvain, Brussels, Belgium

Key Words
Muscle atrophy · Glucocorticoids · Growth factors

Abstract
Background: Many pathological states characterized by muscle atrophy (e.g., sepsis, cachexia, starvation, metabolic acidosis and severe insulinopenia) are associated with an increase in circulating glucocorticoid (GC) levels, suggesting that GC could trigger the muscle atrophy observed in these conditions. GC-induced muscle atrophy results from decreased protein synthesis and increased protein degradation. The inhibitory effect of GCs on protein synthesis is thought to result mainly from the inhibition of the p70 ribosomal S6 protein kinase. The stimulatory effect of GCs on muscle proteolysis results from the activation of two major cellular proteolytic systems: ubiquitin proteasome and lysosomal systems. The decrease in muscle production of insulin-like growth factor I (IGF-I), a muscle anabolic growth factor, could contribute to GC-induced muscle atrophy. By activating the phosphatidylinositol-3-kinase/Akt pathway, IGF-I overrides GC action to stunt muscle atrophy. Evidence also indicates that increased production of myostatin, a catabolic growth factor, could play a critical role in GC-induced muscle atrophy. ***Conclusions:*** Recent progress in understanding the role of growth factors in GC-induced muscle atrophy allows investigation into new therapies to minimize this myopathy.

Introduction

Many pathological conditions characterized by muscle atrophy (e.g., sepsis, cachexia, starvation, metabolic acidosis and severe insulinopenia) are associated with an increase in circulating glucocorticoid (GC) levels, suggesting that this hormone could be a trigger for the muscle atrophy observed in these conditions. In some cases of sepsis, cachexia, starvation and severe insulinopenia, adrenalectomy or treatment with a GC receptor antagonist (i.e., RU-486) attenuates muscle atrophy, indicating that GCs are, in part, responsible for this muscle loss. In addition to GC excess, several other factors, such as poor nutrition, increased cytokine production and being bedridden, may contribute to muscle atrophy observed in these wasting conditions [1]. Typically, skeletal muscle atrophy induced by GCs is characterized by a decrease in the size of fast-twitch, or type II, muscle fibers (particularly IIx and IIb) with little to no impact observed in type I fibers [2]. Therefore, fast-twitch, glycolytic muscles (i.e., tibialis anterior) are more susceptible than oxidative muscles (i.e., soleus) to GC-induced muscle atrophy.

This review is intended to highlight the recent progress made in understanding the growth factor-signaling pathways involved in GC-induced muscle atrophy. Better understanding of the mechanisms of steroid myopathy may lead to new therapeutic options to preserve muscle mass and function in patients receiving high doses of GCs.

KARGER

Fax +41 61 306 12 34
E-Mail karger@karger.ch
www.karger.com

0301–0163/09/0727–0036$26.00/0

Accessible online at:
www.karger.com/hre

Dr. Jean-Paul Thissen
Unité de Diabétologie et Nutrition, Faculté de Médecine
Université Catholique de Louvain, 54 Avenue Hippocrate
BE–1200 Brussels (Belgium)
Tel. +32 2 764 54 69, Fax +32 2 764 54 79, E-Mail jeanpaul.thissen@uclouvain.be

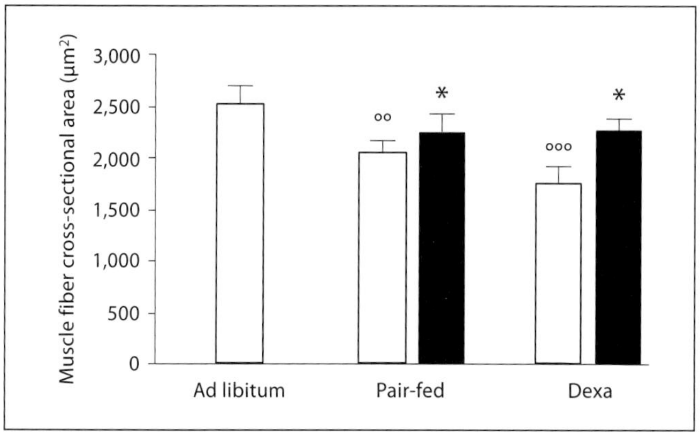

Fig. 1. IGF-I gene electrotransfer prevents muscle atrophy caused by dexamethasone treatment. Tibial anterior muscles were injected and electroporated with a total of 100 μg of pM1 plasmid at a concentration of 1 μg/μl (white column). In pair-fed and dexamethasone-treated rats, contralateral tibial anterior muscles were injected and electroporated with pM1-hIGF-I plasmid at a concentration of 1 μg/μl (black column). Rats were treated with dexamethasone (0.1 mg/kg/day) for 7 days and fiber cross-sectional areas were measured 10 days after DNA injection and electroporation. Results are expressed as mean ± SEM. * $p < 0.05$ vs. contralateral muscle. °° $p < 0.01$, °°° $p < 0.001$ vs. muscle of ad libitum animals. (Reprinted from Schakman et al. [10] with permission from The Endocrine Society. © 2005, The Endocrine Society.)

Changes in Muscle Protein Turnover Caused by GCs

In skeletal muscle, GCs exert their atrophic action by decreasing the rate of protein synthesis and increasing the rate of protein breakdown. Different mechanisms are responsible for the inhibitory effect on protein synthesis. First, GCs inhibit the transport of amino acids into the muscle, limiting protein synthesis. Second, GCs inhibit the stimulatory action of insulin, insulin-like growth factor I (IGF-I) and amino acids (in particular, leucine) on the phosphorylation of the eIF4E-binding protein 1 (4E-BP1) and the p70 ribosomal protein S6 kinase (p70S6K), two factors that play key roles in protein synthesis by controlling the initiation step of mRNA translation. Finally, there is also evidence that GCs cause muscle atrophy by inhibiting myogenesis through the downregulation of myogenin and the degradation of MyoD, two transcription factors required for differentiation of satellite cells into muscle fibers.

The stimulatory effect of GC on muscle proteolysis results from the activation of major cellular proteolytic systems [3], namely the ubiquitin proteasome system (UPS), the lysosomal system (cathepsins) and the calcium-dependent system (calpains). To activate protein degradation, GCs stimulate the expression of several components of the UPS. These components are responsible for either conjugation of ubiquitin to the protein being degraded or protein degradation by the proteasome [4]. This leads to an increased rate of protein ubiquitination and increased proteolytic activities of the proteasome. Since the proteasome does not degrade intact myofibrils, it is thought that actin and myosin need to be dissociated, probably by calpains, from the myofibrils before they can be degraded by the UPS [5]. Finally, some in vivo data also suggest that caspase-3 might be implicated in the myofibrillar protein breakdown induced by GCs. Indeed, in GC-dependent muscle-wasting models, such as severe insulinopenia and chronic renal failure, caspase-3 activity in muscle is increased and inhibition of caspase-3 by Ac-DEVD-CHO (N-acetyl-Asp-Glu-Val-Asp-CHO), a peptide inhibitor, suppresses the accelerated muscle proteolysis. However, the role of GCs in the induction of caspase-3 activity in these models has not yet been elucidated.

Role of IGF-I-Signaling Pathways in GC-Induced Muscle Atrophy

IGF-I

IGF-I is a growth factor that stimulates the development of muscle mass by increasing protein synthesis and myogenesis while decreasing proteolysis and apoptosis [6]. Several observations indicate that decreased muscle IGF-I plays a role in GC-induced muscle atrophy. First, IGF-I inhibits GC-induced proteolysis by downregulating the different proteolytic systems (lysosomal and proteasomal) stimulated by GCs in the myotubes [7, 8]. Second, systemic administration [9] and local overexpression of IGF-I in skeletal muscle prevent GC-induced muscle atrophy [10] (fig. 1). Together, these findings indicate that IGF-I has a dominant effect, overriding GC to shut down catabolism. Evidence also supports the role of several transduction pathways in the antiatrophic effect of IGF-I [11].

Akt

Akt, a serine/threonine kinase activated through phosphorylation by IGF-I, has recently been shown to play a critical role in GC-induced muscle atrophy. Indeed, muscle atrophy induced by GC is associated with a decrease in muscle Akt phosphorylation, and restoration of Akt phosphorylation to normal levels by IGF-I prevents muscle atrophy. More interestingly, overexpression of a

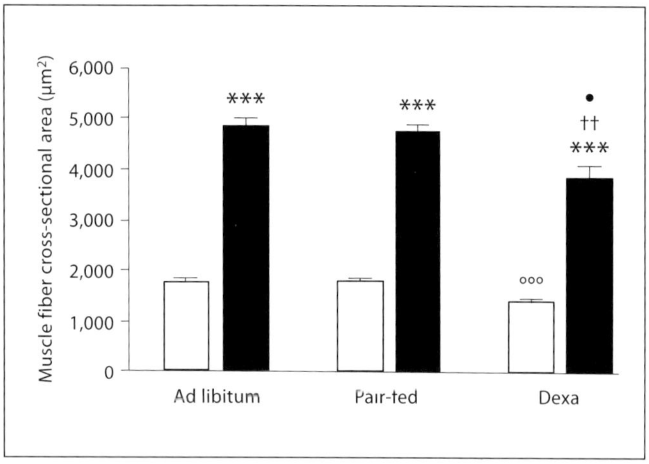

Fig. 2. Constitutively active (ca)Akt muscle overexpression induces a marked fiber hypertrophy and prevents dexamethasone-induced muscle atrophy. caAkt overexpression induced a marked muscle fiber hypertrophy (black column) compared to surrounding untransfected (UT) muscle fibers (white column). Rats were treated with dexamethasone (0.1 mg/kg/day) for 7 days and fiber cross-sectional areas were measured 10 days after DNA injection and electroporation. Results are expressed as mean ± SEM. *** $p < 0.001$ vs. UT muscle fibers of the same muscle. ooo $p < 0.001$ vs. ad libitum UT muscle fibers; †† $p < 0.01$ vs. pair-fed caAkt-transfected muscle fibers; • $p < 0.05$ vs. ad libitum caAkt-transfected muscle fibers. (Reprinted from Schakman et al. [11] with permission from The Endocrine Society. © 2008, The Endocrine Society.)

constitutively active form of Akt overcomes the muscle atrophy caused by GCs [11] (fig. 2). Together, these data support the role of decreased Akt activity in GC-induced muscle atrophy.

mTOR

The inhibition of protein synthesis by GCs results primarily from the inhibition of mTOR, the kinase responsible for the phosphorylation of 4E-BP1 and p70S6K. Repression of mTOR signaling results in a reduction in the initiation phase of mRNA translation with downregulation of protein synthesis. Recent studies have shown that the repression of mTOR signaling in response to GCs is the result of enhanced transcription of REDD1, a repressor of mTOR signaling [12]. mTOR signaling could also be directly inhibited by FOXO, a transcription factor involved in GC-induced muscle atrophy. Whereas the effects of GC on protein synthesis have been explained at the molecular level, comparatively little is known about how these hormones alter anabolic gene expression. Recent studies have identified ATF-4 as an anabolic transcription factor that is repressed by GCs [13]. ATF-4 is required for the activation of a genetic program for the cellular uptake of essential amino acids and the synthesis of nonessential amino acids and aminoacyl-t-RNAs. These observations suggest that GCs inhibit protein synthesis by downregulating ATF-4, limiting intracellular amino acid availability and stimulating REDD1, which inhibits mTOR-mediated protein synthesis.

p70S6K

Inhibition of p70S6K, a target of mTOR that plays a key role in the protein synthesis machinery, is thought to be one of the major mechanisms by which GCs cause muscle atrophy. Phosphorylation of p70S6K is inhibited by GC administration. Prevention of muscle atrophy by IGF-I overexpression in the muscle of GC-treated rats is associated with restoration of p70S6K phosphorylation to normal levels [11]. Decreased p70S6K phosphorylation may result from diminished Akt activity due to GC administration or enhanced transcription of REDD1. Since p70S6K is a target of mTOR, repression of mTOR signaling would also cause repression of p70S6K, resulting in a reduction in the initiation phase of mRNA translation with downregulation of protein synthesis.

Glycogen Synthase Kinase 3β

Glycogen synthase kinase 3β (GSK-3β) is a downstream target of IGF-I signaling that is phosphorylated and inhibited by Akt. GSK-3β may also be involved in the atrophic effect of GC administration since it is known to suppress protein synthesis by inhibiting eukaryotic transcription factor 2B-dependent translation. Inhibition of GSK-3β results in myogenic differentiation and muscle cell hypertrophy and also contributes to the hypertrophic effect of IGF-I on skeletal muscle cells. More interestingly, inhibition of GSK-3β by overexpression of a dominant negative GSK-3β or by pharmacologic inhibitors prevents the proteolysis and cell atrophy caused by GCs in vitro. Furthermore, overexpression of a dominant negative GSK-3β prevents GC-induced muscle atrophy in vivo [11]. The mechanism by which GSK-3β inactivation inhibits muscle protein degradation caused by GCs is not known. However, the observation that inhibition of protein degradation by GSK-3β inhibitors is associated with blockade of the upregulation of several genes characteristic of muscle cell atrophy (atrogenes such as atrogin-1 and MuRF-1 expression) suggests that this reduction in muscle proteolysis is mediated, at least in part, by inhibition of UPS. It is also possible that GSK-3β inactivation inhibits muscle atrophy by blocking the degradation of β-catenin, a transcription factor crucial for physiological muscle growth.

β-Catenin

β-catenin is a small, intracellular, multifunctional protein. In the cytoplasm, the majority of β-catenin is associated with adherens junctions, whereas in the nucleus, β-catenin serves as a transcriptional activator. β-catenin levels are regulated by GSK-3β, which phosphorylates the N-terminal region of β-catenin and induces degradation of β-catenin by UPS. Thus, inhibition of GSK-3β, particularly via Akt phosphorylation, is essential for stabilization and accumulation of β-catenin and its translocation to the nucleus. Recent data suggest a role of β-catenin in GC-induced muscle atrophy and its reversibility by IGF-I. First, muscle atrophy induced by GCs is associated with a large decrease in total β-catenin levels, consistent with the fact that once phosphorylated by GSK-3β, β-catenin is targeted and degraded by the proteasome. Second, the prevention of GC-induced atrophy by IGF-I overexpression is associated with a partial restoration of β-catenin to normal levels. Finally, the overexpression of a stabilized form of β-catenin resistant to proteasomal degradation completely blocks muscle fiber atrophy induced by GCs [11]. The mechanisms by which β-catenin inhibits muscle atrophy are unclear. β-catenin is known to activate transcription of several genes, including some directly implicated in muscle growth. Besides early activation of myogenesis, the β-catenin cascade regulates several genes, including IGFs, PTEN and follistatin, all of which are involved in the regulation of muscle cell size.

FOXO

The role of the transcription factor FOXO in GC-induced muscle cell atrophy was established through different experiments. First, exposure of myotubes to GCs increases FOXO gene expression. Second, both in vitro and in vivo, FOXO overexpression causes muscle cell atrophy together with activation of atrogenes, such as atrogin-1. Finally, overexpression of a dominant negative form of FOXO prevents muscle cell atrophy and atrogin-1 induction caused by GC. Since FOXO, but not atrogin-1, overexpression causes muscle atrophy, FOXO transcription factors likely activate a variety of genes, in addition to atrogin-1, that lead to atrophy. Together, these findings indicate that increased expression of FOXO by GCs activates a gene transcriptional program responsible for triggering muscle atrophy. Among the genes most strongly induced in microarray analyses of muscle atrophy due to a variety of wasting diseases are atrogin-1, MuRF-1, cathepsin-L, PDK4, p21, Gadd45 and 4E-BP1. All of these genes are controlled by FOXO transcription factors. Although these observations support a role of FOXO in GC-induced muscle atrophy, there is no direct in vivo evidence that FOXO is required in this condition.

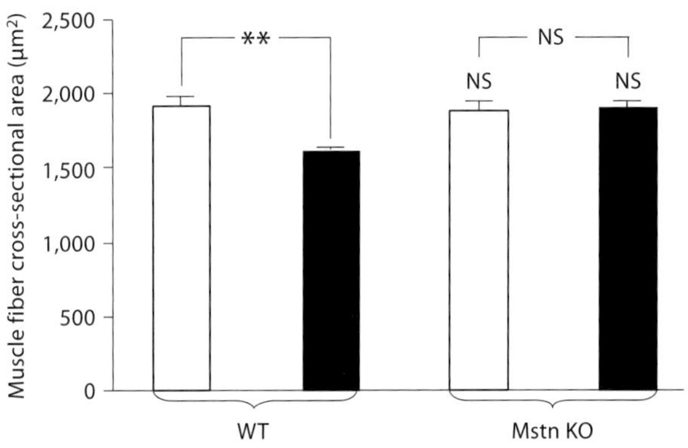

Fig. 3. Deletion of myostatin gene prevents the muscle fiber atrophy induced by dexamethasone treatment. The fiber cross-sectional area was measured on tibialis anterior of wild-type (WT) and myostatin knockout (Mstn KO) mice after 10 days of treatment with dexamethasone (1 mg/kg/day, black column) or saline (white column). Results are expressed as mean ± SEM. ** $p < 0.01$ vs. WT injected with saline; NS = not significant. (Reprinted from Gilson et al. [15] with permission from The Endocrine Society. © 2007, The Endocrine Society.)

Role of Myostatin-Signaling Pathways in GC-Induced Muscle Atrophy

In addition to decreased muscle IGF-I production, GCs also stimulate the production of myostatin (Mstn), a growth factor produced in skeletal muscle that inhibits muscle mass development and causes muscle cell atrophy by downregulating the proliferation and differentiation of satellite cells as well as protein synthesis. Recent evidence indicates that Mstn decreases muscle mass by inhibiting the Akt/mTOR pathway leading to the inhibition of ribosomal protein S6 and activation of 4E-BP1 [14]. For these reasons, increased muscle Mstn has been thought to play a key role in GC-induced muscle atrophy. This hypothesis was recently tested in vivo using Mstn knockout mice. In contrast to wild-type mice, Mstn knockout

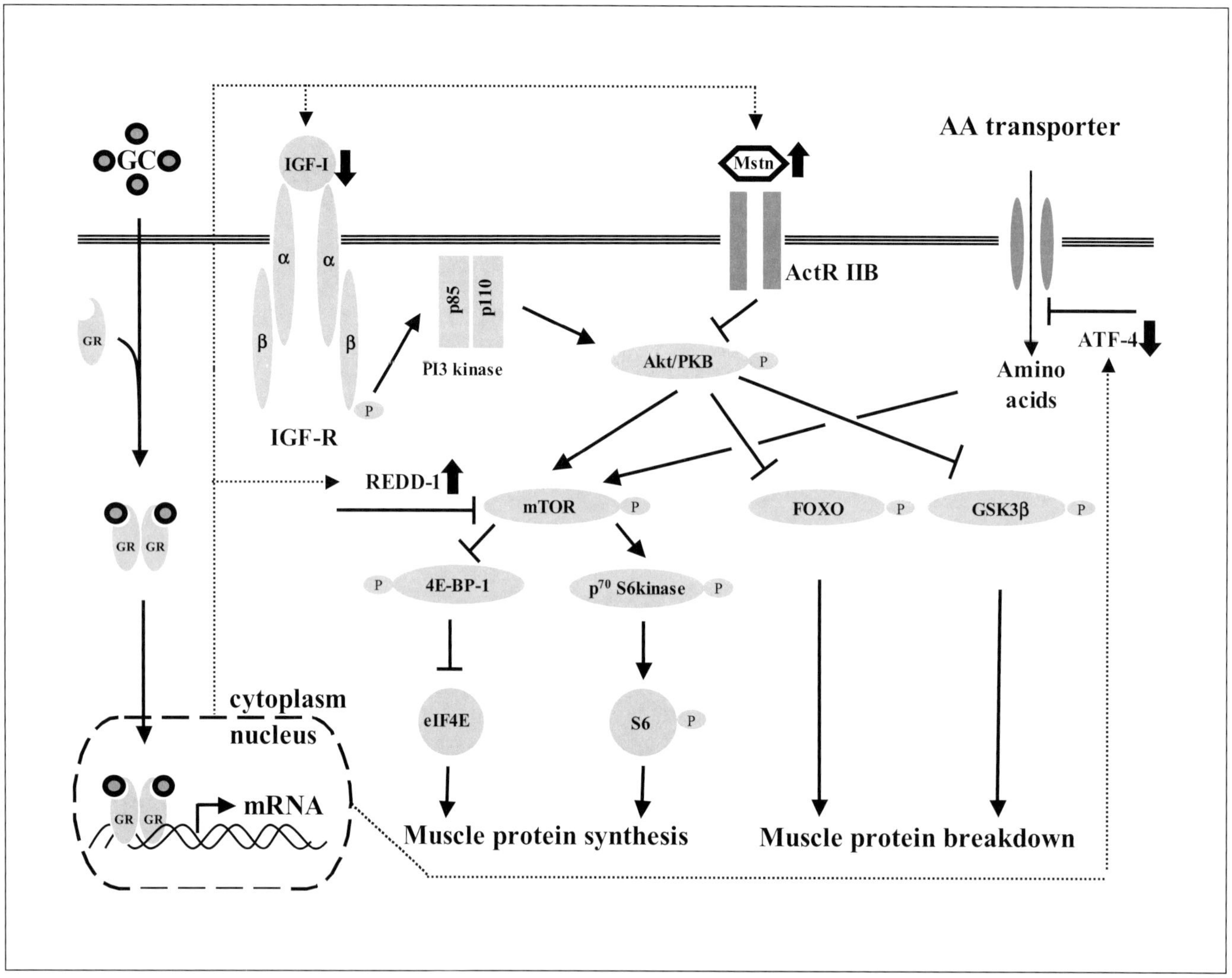

Fig. 4. Signaling pathways involved in glucocorticoid-induced muscle atrophy. Muscle atrophy induced by glucocorticoids is associated with alterations in muscle production of IGF-I and myostatin, two growth factors exhibiting opposite effects on muscle mass development, leading to the inhibition of protein synthesis and stimulation of protein breakdown. These changes in muscle growth factor production occur at similar doses (0.1 to 1 mg/kg/day) to those given in adults and children patients.

mice did not exhibit reduced muscle mass or fiber cross-sectional area following GC treatment [15] (fig. 3). This observation suggests that Mstn is mandatory for the atrophic effects of GCs on skeletal muscle; however, the precise mechanism by which Mstn deletion prevents GC-induced muscle atrophy is unknown. The observation that prevention of muscle atrophy by Mstn deletion is associated with blockade of the upregulation of atrogene expression and proteasomal activity following GC administration suggests that the protective effect on muscle mass is due partly to the inhibition of muscle proteolysis [15]. Thus, in addition to stimulating IGF-I production, inhibition of Mstn may be useful in reversing the catabolic effects of GC excess.

Conclusions

GCs appear to play a crucial role in muscle atrophy observed in various pathological conditions (fig. 4). Both decreased protein synthesis and increased protein degradation contribute to this muscle atrophy. Different intracellular mediators, such as Akt, mTOR, GSK-3β, β-catenin, FOXO, REDD1 and ATF4, are involved in the muscle catabolic and antianabolic effects of GCs. IGF-I stimulation or Mstn blockade constitutes some of the most promising future therapeutic approaches to prevent GC-induced muscle atrophy. Although many unanswered questions remain, understanding the cellular basis of GC-induced skeletal muscle atrophy will enable rational development of therapeutic interventions to minimize the debilitating effects of GCs on skeletal muscle.

Acknowledgments

The work of the authors is supported by grants from the Fund for Scientific Medical Research (Belgium), the National Fund for Scientific Research (Belgium), the Association Française contre les Myopathies (France) and the Fonds Spéciaux de Recherche (Université Catholique de Louvain, Belgium).

Disclosure Statement

The authors have nothing to disclose.

References

1 Schakman O, Gilson H, Thissen JP: Mechanisms of glucocorticoid-induced myopathy. J Endocrinol 2008;197:1–10.
2 Dekhuijzen PN, Gayan-Ramirez G, Bisschop A, de Bock V, Dom R, Decramer M: Corticosteroid treatment and nutritional deprivation cause a different pattern of atrophy in rat diaphragm. J Appl Physiol 1995;78:629–637.
3 Hasselgren PO: Glucocorticoids and muscle catabolism. Curr Opin Clin Nutr Metab Care 1999;2:201–205.
4 Bodine SC, Latres E, Baumhueter S, Lai VKM, Nunez L, Clarke BA, Poueymirou WT, Panaro FJ, Na EQ, Dharmarajan K, Pan ZQ, Valenzuela DM, DeChiara TM, Stitt TN, Yancopoulos GD, Glass DJ: Identification of ubiquitin ligases required for skeletal muscle atrophy. Science 2001;294:1704–1708.
5 Hasselgren PO, Fischer JE: Muscle cachexia: current concepts of intracellular mechanisms and molecular regulation. Ann Surg 2001;233:9–17.
6 Florini JR, Ewton DZ, Coolican SA: Growth hormone and the insulin-like growth factor system in myogenesis. Endocr Rev 1996;17:481–517.
7 Dehoux M, Van Beneden R, Pasko N, Lause P, Verniers J, Underwood L, Ketelslegers JM, Thissen JP: Role of the insulin-like growth factor I decline in the induction of atrogin-1/MAFbx during fasting and diabetes. Endocrinology 2004;145:4806–4812.
8 Latres E, Amini AR, Amini AA, Griffiths J, Martin FJ, Wei Y, Lin HC, Yancopoulos GD, Glass DJ: Insulin-like growth factor-1 (IGF-1) inversely regulates atrophy-induced genes via the phosphatidylinositol 3-kinase/Akt/mammalian target of rapamycin (PI3K/Akt/mTOR) pathway. J Biol Chem 2005;280:2737–2744.
9 Fournier M, Huang ZS, Li H, Da X, Cercek B, Lewis MI: Insulin-like growth factor-I prevents corticosteroid-induced diaphragm muscle atrophy in emphysematous hamsters. Am J Physiol Regul Integr Comp Physiol 2003;285:R34–R43.
10 Schakman O, Gilson H, de Coninck V, Lause P, Verniers J, Havaux X, Ketelslegers JM, Thissen JP: Insulin-like growth factor-I gene transfer by electroporation prevents skeletal muscle atrophy in glucocorticoid-treated rats. Endocrinology 2005;146:1789–1797.
11 Schakman O, Kalista S, Bertrand L, Lause P, Verniers J, Ketelslegers JM, Thissen JP: Role of Akt/GSK-3beta/beta-catenin transduction pathway in the muscle anti-atrophy action of insulin-like growth factor-I in glucocorticoid-treated rats. Endocrinology 2008;149:3900–3908.
12 Wang H, Kubica N, Ellisen LW, Jefferson LS, Kimball SR: Dexamethasone represses signaling through the mammalian target of rapamycin in muscle cells by enhancing expression of REDD1. J Biol Chem 2006;281:39128–39134.
13 Adams CM: Role of the transcription factor ATF4 in the anabolic actions of insulin and the anti-anabolic actions of glucocorticoids. J Biol Chem 2007;282:16744–16753.
14 Amirouche A, Durieux AC, Banzet S, Koulmann N, Bonnefoy R, Mouret C, Bigard X, Peinnequin A, Freyssenet D: Down-regulation of Akt/mTOR signaling pathway in response to myostatin overexpression in skeletal muscle. Endocrinology 2009;150:286–294.
15 Gilson H, Schakman O, Combaret L, Lause P, Grobet L, Attaix D, Ketelslegers JM, Thissen JP: Myostatin gene deletion prevents glucocorticoid-induced muscle atrophy. Endocrinology 2007;148:452–460.

HORMONE
RESEARCH

Horm Res 2009;72(suppl 1):42–47
DOI: 10.1159/000229763

Published online: November 27, 2009

Promoting Growth in Chronic Inflammatory Disease: Lessons from Studies of the Growth Plate

S.F. Ahmed[a] L. Sävendahl[b]

[a]Bone and Endocrine Research Group, Division of Developmental Medicine, University of Glasgow, Royal Hospital for Sick Children, Glasgow, UK; [b]Department of Woman and Child Health, Pediatric Endocrinology Unit, Astrid Lindgren Children's Hospital, Karolinska Institute, Stockholm, Sweden

Key Words
Growth · Children · Inflammatory disease · Glucocorticoids

Abstract

Background: Growth disorders are commonly observed in children with chronic inflammatory disease. It is likely that these disorders are mediated by a combination of factors, including the disease process and its treatment (with drugs such as glucocorticoids [GCs]). These factors affect the growth hormone-insulin-like growth factor I (IGF-I) axis, which is crucial for promoting linear growth at the level of the growth plate. Recent advances in our knowledge of the effects of GCs and proinflammatory cytokines on the growth plate have led to an improved understanding of the biological rationale for the use of growth-promoting therapy in children with chronic inflammatory disease and concurrent growth retardation. ***Conclusions:*** Both GCs and proinflammatory cytokines can adversely affect a number of components of growth plate chondrogenesis, and these effects can be ameliorated by raising local IGF-I exposure. However, this intervention does not lead to complete normalization of the growth plate. In children with chronic inflammation, the cornerstone of improving growth remains the judicious use of GCs while ensuring effective control of the disease process.

The Growth Plate

Growth of long bones occurs at the growth plate, a thin layer of cartilage that separates the epiphysis from the metaphysis. The growth plate is a highly complex, spatially polarized structure that consists of 3 layers: the stem cell zone, the proliferative zone and the hypertrophic zone. Chondrocytes in the stem cell zone are recruited to start active proliferation and then undergo differentiation, which is followed by apoptosis and eventually mineralization. Many systemic hormones, including growth hormone (GH), insulin-like growth factor I (IGF-I), insulin, thyroid hormone, glucocorticoids (GCs) and sex steroids, regulate longitudinal bone growth. In both mice and humans with inactivating mutations in the GH receptor, increased circulating IGF-I can markedly improve linear bone growth, supporting a role for circulating IGF-I in modulating longitudinal bone growth [1, 2]. GH can also stimulate bone growth by a local action on the growth plate. Injection of GH into the tibial growth plate accelerates longitudinal growth when compared with the vehicle-injected contralateral growth plate [3]. Part of the local action of GH on the growth plate may be mediated by increased local production of IGF-I, which then acts in a paracrine-autocrine fashion to increase chondrogenesis [4, 5].

KARGER

Fax +41 61 306 12 34
E-Mail karger@karger.ch
www.karger.com

0301–0163/09/0727–0042$26.00/0

Accessible online at:
www.karger.com/hre

Dr. Lars Sävendahl
Department of Woman and Child Health, Pediatric Endocrinology Unit
Astrid Lindgren Children's Hospital, Karolinska Institute
SE–17176 Stockholm (Sweden)
Tel. +46 8 5177 2369, Fax +46 8 5177 5128, E-Mail lars.savendahl@kbh.ki.se

Effects of GCs on Growth

Long-term treatment with GCs suppresses longitudinal bone growth through a number of mechanisms. High-dose GC therapy attenuates physiological GH by increasing somatostatin tone. GH response to GH stimulation tests may be reversibly impaired in some cases of steroid exposure. The finding that some children with growth failure caused by long-term GC therapy have normal GH and IGF-I levels indicates the possible end-organ insensitivity for these hormones. GC-induced growth failure may also be due to direct effects on the growth plate. GC receptors are expressed by growth plate chondrocytes [6], and growth retardation induced by dexamethasone is associated with increased chondrocyte apoptosis at the growth plate [7]. When administered topically – even as eye drops – GCs may cause growth retardation and reduced bone mineral density [8, 9]. Interestingly, infusion of dexamethasone into the growth plate has resulted in local inhibition of longitudinal bone growth [10], and it is also believed to disrupt the growth plate vasculature. Chondrocytes exposed to GCs show reduced proliferation, a reversible, prolonged resting period, marked reduction in matrix synthesis and increased rates of apoptosis [11, 12]. In addition, GC-induced apoptosis is mediated through activation of caspases and suppression of the Akt-phosphatidylinositol 3-kinase (PI3K) signaling pathway [13, 14]. In vitro studies suggest that local somatotrophic action of GH and IGF-I may be affected by a number of different mechanisms, including alterations in the activity of the GH-binding protein, downregulation of GH-receptor expression and binding capacity and reduced local IGF-I production and activity. GC-induced reduction of growth in vitro is also reported to be associated with reduced growth of the mineralizing zone of the growth plate [12]. Interestingly, there was no notable growth-sparing effect with alternate-day administration of GCs [12].

Addressing the GC Insult as a Means of Promoting Growth

Mitigating the insult induced by GC administration requires cautious use of these potent drugs. More direct administration, such as intra-articular injections, may avoid the use of long-term systemic doses. Early use of steroid-sparing immunomodulator therapy is becoming more commonplace; however, given that the majority of efficacy data involves the use of GCs, clinicians often rely on the use of these drugs as primary therapy. Selective GC-receptor modulators are a novel class of drugs that may exert sufficient anti-inflammatory effects without the growth-inhibiting effects of traditional GCs. In vitro studies at the level of the growth plate suggest that these drugs have less of a growth-inhibiting effect than dexamethasone at equipotent anti-inflammatory doses [15]. GH treatment may result in rescued growth and partially prevent the negative effects of GCs on growth plate chondrogenesis in uremic rats [16]. In this animal model, GH administration stimulated proliferative activity and hypertrophy in the growth plate chondrocytes [16]. In the mouse metatarsal model of longitudinal growth, which has not shown any notable response to GH administration, exposure to IGF-I reversed the growth-inhibiting effects of GCs (fig. 1) [12]. However, the potential for GCs to inhibit bone growth persisted, despite concomitant administration of IGF-I. It is possible that GCs may inhibit downstream signaling of the IGF-I receptor through the PI3K pathway [14]. In addition, the IGF-I-mediated improvement that was observed in the mouse model occurred at the expense of altering the balance among the proliferating, hypertrophic and mineralizing zones within the metatarsal (fig. 1) [12].

Cytokine Effects on Growth

The complex interaction of molecular signals involved in growth plate chondrogenesis is often dysregulated during chronic illnesses and results in growth failure. The principal events responsible for this are inflammation, protein/calorie deprivation, uremia/metabolic acidosis, GC administration and an impaired GH–IGF-I axis. Elevated levels of circulating interleukin (IL)-6 have been observed in children with chronic inflammatory disease. In many cases, these patients show reduced circulating IGF-I levels with unchanged GH levels. The proinflammatory cytokine tumor necrosis factor alpha (TNFα) is also elevated in children with juvenile idiopathic arthritis (JIA). TNF-transgenic mice, which overexpress TNFα, show growth retardation; however, alterations in the GH–IGF-I axis have not been examined in this transgenic model. In contrast, IL-1β treatment is known to reduce plasma levels of both IGF-I and the acid-labile subunit.

The effect of proinflammatory cytokines, particularly IL-6, IL-1β and TNFα, on chondrocytes has been comprehensively studied in vitro. However, investigations have predominantly focused on the effects of cytokines

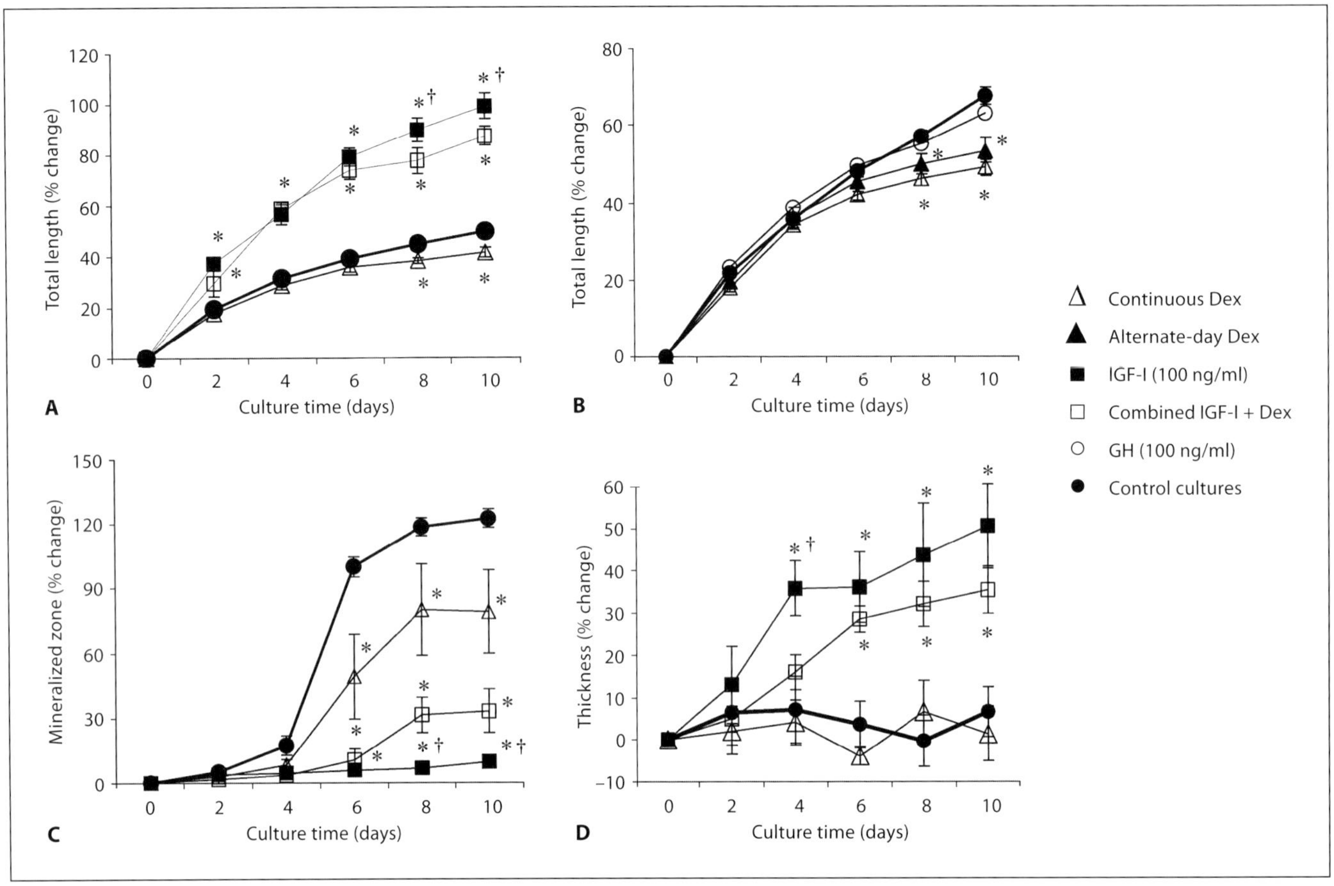

Fig. 1. The effects of dexamethasone (Dex), GH and IGF-I on the growth of fetal mouse metatarsals in culture. **A** Continuous Dex at 10^{-6} M caused a significant decrease in linear growth from day 8, whereas IGF-I and IGF-I + Dex had significant stimulatory effects from day 2. **B** Effects of GH (100 ng/ml) and continuous and alternate-day Dex on total length. GH had no significant effects on total length. However, both continuous and alternate-day Dex caused a significant decrease in length from day 8 ($p < 0.05$). **C** Effects of Dex, IGF-I, and IGF-I + Dex on the length of the mineralized zone. In the control metatarsals, mineralization increased from day 4. All treatments caused a significant reduction in mineralization from day 6. IGF-I-treated bones were the least mineralized, whereas Dex and IGF-I + Dex effects were intermediate. **D** Effects of Dex, IGF-I, and IGF-I + Dex on metatarsal thickness. Both IGF-I and IGF-I + Dex caused a significant increase in the metatarsal thickness from day 4 and 6, respectively. Results shown in **A**, **B**, and **D** were obtained from the same cultures, whereas the data shown in **B** were from a separate experiment. All data are expressed as the mean ± SEM; * $p < 0.05$ compared with control; † significance of IGF-I compared with IGF-I/Dex ($p < 0.05$). (Adapted from Mushtaq et al. [12] with permission from The Endocrine Society. ©2004, The Endocrine Society.)

on articular chondrocytes rather than on growth plate chondrocytes. Local injection of adenovirus into the knee joints in rodents has resulted in infection of the chondrocytes in the growth plate, particularly the hypertrophic chondrocytes, suggesting that local joint inflammation may have harmful effects on adjacent growth plates (fig. 2) [17, 18]. Our knowledge about cytokine effects on human growth plate cartilage is limited. Most in vitro studies have concentrated on IL-6, IL-1β and TNFα; however, it is becoming increasingly clear that chronic inflammatory disease is associated with a variable level of alteration in many pro- and anti-inflammatory cytokines [19, 20]. Both IL-1β and TNFα inhibit growth plate chondrocyte differentiation, increase apoptosis and inhibit cartilage-specific proteoglycan synthesis in ATDC5 murine growth plate cells as well as the rodent metatarsal model (fig. 3) [21, 22]. On the other hand, IL-1β has also been shown to increase DNA synthesis in growth plate chondrocytes [23], which may be the mechanism for the excessive endochondral bone growth observed in the affected limbs

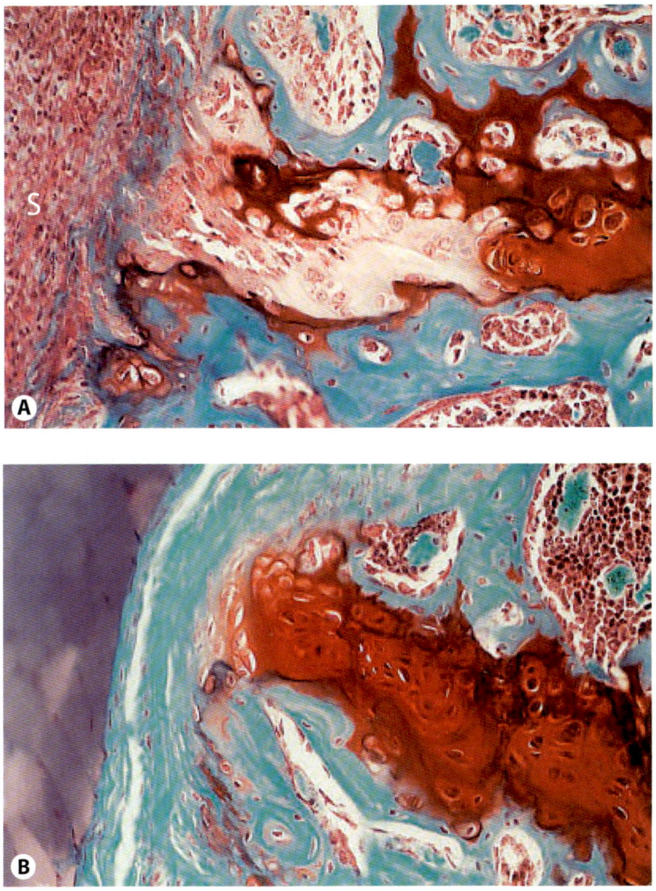

2

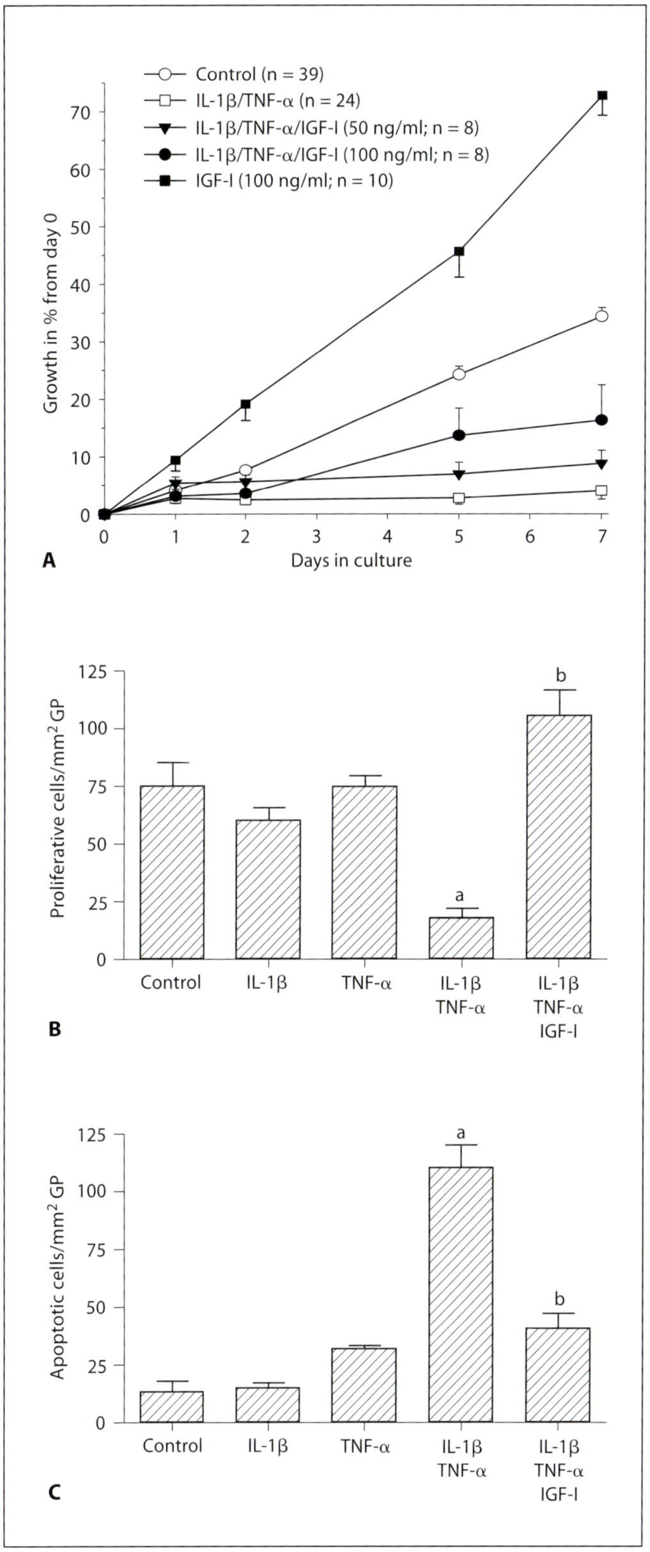

3

Fig. 2. Joint inflammation leads to proteoglycan depletion and disorganization of the adjacent growth plate. Growth plate damage was induced by injection of the adenoviral murine oncostatin M vector (AdMuOSM) into the knee joint of wild-type mice. **A** Proteoglycan depletion and disorganization of the growth plate on day 7 after injection of AdMuOSM. S = Inflamed synovium. **B** Normal growth plate on day 7 after injection of control vector. (Safranin O stained; original magnification ×200; adapted from de Hooge et al. [18] with permission of the American College of Rheumatology.)

Fig. 3. Effect of IGF-I on proinflammatory cytokine-induced growth retardation. **A** IGF-I (50 or 100 ng/ml) partially rescued cultured fetal rat metatarsal bones from cytokine-induced suppression of longitudinal bone growth. The cytokines, IL-1β and TNF-α (IL-1β/TNF-α; 10 ng/ml each), were added to all groups except the control and IGF-I only groups. Substances were included in the culture medium from day 0. **B** and **C** show the effects of IL-1β (10 ng/ml) and TNF-α (10 ng/ml) when added individually or in combination at the same concentrations to fetal rat metatarsal bones kept in culture for 7 days. IGF-I (100 ng/ml) was capable of rescuing chondrocyte proliferation (**B**) and preventing apoptosis (**C**) induced by the combined treatment with IL-1 and TNF-α (10 ng/ml each). Results are expressed as number of positive cells per mm^2 growth plate surface area (mean ± SE). Evaluation of cell proliferation with BrdU immuno-labeling (**B**) and apoptosis by TUNEL immunohistochemistry (**C**). ^{a} $p < 0.001$ vs. control; ^{b} $p < 0.001$ vs. IL-β/TNF-α. (Adapted from Martensson et al. [21] with permission of the American Society for Bone and Mineral Research.)

of children with oligoarticular JIA. Proinflammatory cytokines also have additive or synergistic effects such that, when combined, more severely hinder longitudinal growth in the rodent metatarsal model [21, 22]. Furthermore, the duration of exposure to proinflammatory cytokines in the culture model is important: while a short exposure to cytokines is associated with minimal reduction in long-term growth, longer exposure leads to a dramatic, irreversible reduction in growth [22].

The cellular mechanisms through which cytokines act on the growth plate have yet to be elucidated, but may include the downregulation of key chondrocyte regulatory factors, such as expression of *Sox9* gene, inhibition of IGF-I signaling and interference with GH signaling. IL-1β and TNFα can induce the expression of a suppressor of cytokine signaling proteins that downregulate cytokine signaling and alter GH signaling. IL-1β may also inhibit IGF-I–induced bone growth through the PI3K pathway [14].

Addressing the Cytokine Insult as a Means of Promoting Growth

Addressing the primary disease remains the cornerstone for optimizing the growth of children with chronic inflammatory diseases, including JIA. The recent introduction of anti-TNF agents has revolutionized the treatment of JIA. Anti-TNF treatment leads to a significant decrease in disease activity in adult rheumatoid arthritis [24] and in JIA [25]. Etanercept is a recombinant fusion protein that acts as a soluble receptor through competitive inhibition with the TNF receptor on the cell surface. The result is a reduction in the TNF-driven inflammation that plays a key role in the arthritic process. In a mixed population of seven prepubertal and pubertal patients with refractory JIA and growth retardation, anti-TNF therapy was associated with growth resumption [26]. A larger study of 71 prepubertal and pubertal patients with JIA showed similar results [27]. In a more recent study, etanercept improved linear growth and reduced the need for intra-articular GC injections in a majority of prepubertal and pubertal patients with JIA not responding to conventional therapy [28]. It is unclear whether the sole growth-promoting effect of these drugs is through steroid sparing or direct effects on cytokines at the level of the growth plate. MacRae and colleagues recently showed that the inhibitory effect of serum and synovial fluid collected from children with JIA and containing a wide range of cytokines was not ameliorated by a combination of anti-IL-1β, TNFα and IL-6 antibodies, even at high concentrations [19]. In the rodent metatarsal model, which does not respond to GH stimulation, IGF-I administration ameliorates cytokine-induced growth retardation and reduces the level of chondrocyte apoptosis [21]. However, longitudinal growth remained stunted despite IGF-I administration [21].

Conclusions

The development of abnormal growth patterns in children with inflammatory diseases such as JIA may be mediated by proinflammatory cytokines and GCs through both systemic effects on the GH–IGF-I axis and local effects at the level of the growth plate. The effects at the growth plate level may partly involve the GH–IGF-I axis. Specific immunomodulatory therapy that targets the actions of TNFα has proven at least partially effective at rescuing linear growth in many children with JIA. The minority of patients with JIA who do not respond to anti-TNF treatment may be candidates for therapeutic agents that target other proinflammatory cytokines and also for GH intervention. Although GH treatment has been shown to rescue linear growth in some patients with JIA, it is unknown whether GH is capable of rescuing growth in those patients with JIA who have not responded to anticytokine therapy. Further experimental and clinical studies are needed to explore these and other new potential treatment strategies that optimize linear growth in patients who do not respond to conventional therapy.

Disclosure Statement

S.F.A. declares no conflict of interest. L.S. declares no conflict of interest.

References

1 Guevara-Aguirre J, Rosenbloom AL, Vasconez O, Martinez V, Gargosky SE, Allen L, Rosenfeld RG: Two-year treatment of growth hormone (GH) receptor deficiency with recombinant insulin-like growth factor I in 22 children: comparison of two dosage levels and to GH-treated GH deficiency. J Clin Endocrinol Metab 1997;82:629–633.

2 Sims NA, Clement-Lacroix P, Da Ponte F, Bouali Y, Binart N, Moriggl R, Goffin V, Coschigano K, Gaillard-Kelly M, Kopchick J, Baron R, Kelly PA: Bone homeostasis in growth hormone receptor-null mice is restored by IGF-I but independent of Stat5. J Clin Invest 2000;106:1095–1103.

3 Isaksson OG, Jansson JO, Gause IA: Growth hormone stimulates longitudinal bone growth directly. Science 1982;216:1237–1239.
4 Isgaard J, Moller C, Isaksson OG, Nilsson A, Mathews LS, Norstedt G: Regulation of insulin-like growth factor messenger ribonucleic acid in rat growth plate by growth hormone. Endocrinology 1988;122:1515–1520.
5 Schlechter NL, Russell SM, Spencer EM, Nicoll CS: Evidence suggesting that the direct growth-promoting effect of growth hormone on cartilage in vivo is mediated by local production of somatomedin. Proc Natl Acad Sci USA 1986;83:7932–7934.
6 Silvestrini G, Ballanti P, Patacchioli FR, Mocetti P, Di Grezia R, Wedard BM, Angelucci L, Bonucci E: Evaluation of apoptosis and the glucocorticoid receptor in the cartilage growth plate and metaphyseal bone cells of rats after high-dose treatment with corticosterone. Bone 2000;26:33–42.
7 Chrysis D, Ritzen EM, Sävendahl L: Growth retardation induced by dexamethasone is associated with increased apoptosis of the growth plate chondrocytes. J Endocrinol 2003;176:331–337.
8 Kugelberg M, Shafiei K, Ohlsson C, Sävendahl L, Zetterström C: Glucocorticoid eye drops inhibit growth in the newborn rabbit. Acta Paediatr 2005;94:1096–1101.
9 Kugelberg M, Shafiei K, Ohlsson C, Zetterström C, Sävendahl L: Reduced bone mineral density and radial bone growth in young rabbits treated with dexamethasone eye drops. Horm Res 2005;63:165–170.
10 Baron J, Huang Z, Oerter KE, Bacher JD, Cutler GB Jr: Dexamethasone acts locally to inhibit longitudinal bone growth in rabbits. Am J Physiol 1992;263:489–492.
11 Mushtaq T, Seawright E, Farquharson C, Ahmed SF: Glucocorticoid effects on chondrogenesis, differentiation and apoptosis on the ATDC5 chondrocyte cell line. J Endocrinol 2002;175:705–713.
12 Mushtaq T, Bijman P, Ahmed SF, Farquharson C: Insulin like growth factor-I augments chondrocyte hypertrophy and reverses glucocorticoid mediated growth retardation in fetal mice metatarsal cultures. Endocrinology 2004;145:2478–2486.
13 Chrysis D, Zaman F, Chagin AS, Takigawa M, Sävendahl L: Dexamethasone induces apoptosis in proliferative chondrocytes through activation of caspases and suppression of the Akt-(PI3K) signaling pathway. Endocrinology 2005;146:1391–1397.
14 MacRae VE, Mushtaq T, Ahmed SF, Farquharson C: IGF-I signaling in bone growth: inhibitory actions of dexamethasone and IL-1beta. Growth Horm IGF Res 2007;17:435–439.
15 Owen HC, Miner JN, Ahmed SF, Farquharson C: The growth plate sparing effects of the selective glucocorticoid receptor modulator, AL-438. Mol Cell Endocrinol 2007;264:164–170.
16 Barbosa APF, Silva JDP, Fonseca EC, Lopez PM, Fernandes MBC, Balduino A, Duarte MEL: Response of the growth plate of uremic rats to human growth hormone and corticosteroids. Braz J Med Biol Res 2007;40:1101–1109.
17 Joronen K, Ala-aho R, Majuri ML, Alenius H, Kähäri VM, Vuorio E: Adenovirus mediated intra-articular expression of collagenase-3 (MMP-13) induces inflammatory arthritis in mice. Ann Rheum Dis 2004;63:656–664.
18 de Hooge AS, van de Loo FA, Bennink MB, Arntz OJ, Fiselier TJ, Franssen MJ, Joosten LA, Van Lent PL, Richards CD, van den Berg WB: Growth plate damage, a feature of juvenile idiopathic arthritis, can be induced by adenoviral gene transfer of oncostatin M: a comparative study in gene-deficient mice. Arthritis Rheum 2003;48:1750–1761.
19 MacRae VE, Wong SC, Smith W, Gracie A, McInnes I, Galea P, Gardner-Medwin J, Farquharson C, Ahmed SF: Cytokine profiling and in-vitro studies of metatarsal growth using biological fluids from children with juvenile idiopathic arthritis. Clin Endocrinol (Oxford) 2007;67:442–448.
20 Wong SC, MacRae VE, Smith W, Gracie A, McInnes I, Galea P, Gardner-Medwin J, Ahmed SF: Inflammatory cytokines in juvenile idiopathic arthritis: effects on physical growth and the insulin-like-growth factor axis. Growth Horm IGF Res 2008;18:369–378.
21 Martensson K, Chrysis D, Sävendahl L: Interleukin-1 beta and TNF-alpha act in synergy to inhibit longitudinal growth in fetal rat metatarsal bones. J Bone Miner Res 2004;19:1805–1812.
22 MacRae VE, Farquharson C, Ahmed SF: The restricted potential for recovery of growth plate chondrogenesis and longitudinal bone growth following exposure to pro-inflammatory cytokines. J Endocrinol 2006;189:319–328.
23 Söder O, Madsen K: Stimulation of chondrocyte DNA synthesis by interleukin-1. Br J Rheumatol 1988;27:21–26.
24 Elliott MJ, Maini RN, Feldmann M, Kalden JR, Antoni C, Smolen JS, Leeb B, Breedveld FC, Macfarlane JD, Bijl H, Woody JN: Randomised double-blind comparison of chimeric monoclonal antibody to tumour necrosis factor alpha (cA2) versus placebo in rheumatoid arthritis. Lancet 1994;344:1105–1110.
25 Lovell DJ, Giannini EH, Reiff A, Cawkwell GD, Silverman ED, Nocton JJ, Stein LD, Gedalia A, Ilowite NT, Wallace CA, Whitmore J, Finck BK: Etanercept in children with polyarticular juvenile rheumatoid arthritis. Pediatric Rheumatology Collaborative Study Group. N Engl J Med 2000;342:763–769.
26 Schmeling H, Seliger E, Horneff G: Growth reconstitution in juvenile idiopathic arthritis treated with etanercept. Clin Exp Rheumatol 2003;21:779–784.
27 Tynjala P, Lahdenne P, Vahasalo P, Kautiainen H, Honkanen V: Impact of anti-TNF treatment on growth in severe juvenile idiopathic arthritis. Ann Rheum Dis 2006;65:1044–1049.
28 Fernandéz P, Hansen JB, Andersson U, Sävendahl S, Hagelberg S: Etanercept treatment improves longitudinal growth in prepubertal children with juvenile idiopathic arthritis. J Rheumatol 2007;34:2481–2485.

HORMONE RESEARCH

Horm Res 2009;72(suppl 1):48–54
DOI: 10.1159/000229764

Published online: November 27, 2009

Can Growth Hormone Counteract the Catabolic Effects of Steroids?

Nelly Mauras

Division of Endocrinology, Nemours Children's Clinic, Jacksonville, Fla., USA

Key Words
Growth hormone · IGF-I · Catabolic effects

Abstract
Background: Chronic administration of glucocorticosteroids (GCs) can have significant catabolic effects in vivo in a host of metabolic systems, including amino acid metabolism, skeletal muscle, bone and linear growth. GCs inhibit protein synthesis and increase protein breakdown at the skeletal muscle and whole-body level and impair growth hormone (GH) secretion and action. Conversely, GH and insulin-like growth factor I (IGF-I) are potent protein-anabolic and growth-promoting agents in vitro and in vivo. This review summarizes both the catabolic effects of GCs and the anabolic and metabolic effects of GH and IGF-I. ***Conclusions:*** Both GH and IGF-I may decrease the catabolic effects of chronic steroid use in humans, particularly by enhancing lean body mass accrual and, in children, by increasing linear growth.

The Catabolic Effects of Glucocorticoids on Protein Metabolism and Body Composition

The catabolic effects of chronic steroid use are due to their interaction with multiple systems. Chronic glucocorticoid (GC) use inhibits the transport of amino acids into skeletal muscle. It also inhibits the stimulatory actions of insulin-like growth factor I (IGF-I), insulin and amino acids per se on the phosphorylation of eIF4EBP1 and S6K1, factors that play key roles in protein synthesis by controlling the initiation of mRNA translation. GCs also repress ATF-4, a transcription factor needed for the muscle uptake of amino acids [1]. Chronic GC administration also causes muscle atrophy by inhibiting myogenesis through the downregulation of myogenin, a critical transcription factor for the differentiation of satellite cells into muscle fibers [1].

Chronic steroid use also stimulates proteolysis through different mechanisms including the activation of FOXO, a transcription factor that appears to activate a gene transcriptional program responsible for triggering muscle atrophy [1]. Also, GCs, at least in vitro, stimulate glycogen synthase kinase 3β, which in turn inhibits other transcription factors involved in mRNA translation. At the whole-body level, studies using isotope-labeled infusions of leucine, an essential amino acid, have shown that GCs inhibit leucine uptake and potently stimulate whole body proteolysis [2].

Local production of IGF-I, which stimulates muscle mass development, protein synthesis and myogenesis, is also inhibited by chronic GC use. In contrast, myostatin, a growth factor that inhibits muscle mass development (including proliferation and differentiation), is stimulated by chronic use of GCs [1]. Hence, when given in pharmacological doses and for prolonged periods, GCs are highly catabolic agents on protein systems.

These factors affecting protein synthesis and degradation, as well as muscle protein function, are largely responsible for the loss of lean body mass and strength that

KARGER

Fax +41 61 306 12 34
E-Mail karger@karger.ch
www.karger.com

0301–0163/09/0727–0048$26.00/0

Accessible online at:
www.karger.com/hre

Prof. Nelly Mauras
Division of Endocrinology
Nemours Children's Clinic, 807 Children's Way
Jacksonville, FL 32207 (USA)
Tel. +1 904 697 3674, Fax +1 904 697 3948, E-Mail nmauras@nemours.org

are observed with chronic GC use. In humans, chronic hypercortisolemia, whether endogenous or exogenous, also causes a marked increase in adiposity, particularly intra-abdominally [3], thereby negatively influencing body composition (i.e., lesser lean body mass and greater fat mass).

Anabolic Effects of Growth Hormone and IGF-I

Growth hormone (GH) has important metabolic functions in vivo, many of which are mediated via IGF-I. IGF-I has both GH-like actions and insulin-like actions and its in vivo effects depend on dosing, length of use and even route of administration. GH has proliferative, inhibitory and metabolic effects. The mechanisms of hormonal secretion and action of GH have been extensively reviewed [4]. GH interacts with two GH receptors (GHRs) at two different binding sites in GH-sensitive cells. This interaction activates a complex signaling transduction cascade of events, including Janus kinase and STAT phosphorylation, which results in the generation of IGF-I. This process triggers the proliferative effects of GH through the mitogen-activated protein kinase system, causing stimulation of transcription factors and ultimately resulting in linear growth. The inhibitory effects of GH, on the other hand, are mediated in part by suppressors of cytokine signaling [5], mutations of which result in exaggerated growth [6]. Some of the metabolic effects of GH, however, result from activation of the insulin receptor substrate and phosphatidyl inositol 3 kinases; these are independent of IGF-I generation.

Because it has approximately 8% equipotency with insulin, IGF-I works through both the type 1 IGF-I receptor and the insulin receptor [7]. Even though insulin is about 100-fold more potent than IGF-I in activating its own receptor, IGF-I can activate the insulin receptor in supraphysiologic or pharmacologic concentrations. This causes the known hypoglycemic effects of IGF-I (discussed below) [8]. The hypoglycemic effects of IGF-I are also mediated by activation of its own IGF-I receptor [9].

Effects on Protein Metabolism

An extensive body of data shows that both GH and IGF-I have potent protein-anabolic effects in humans [10]. We administered GH and IGF-I for 2 months each in short-term studies of severely GH-deficient adults. Our results showed that both had significant anabolic effects, although GH appeared to be more potent than IGF-I in the doses used [11]. Both hormones increased lean body mass and decreased fat mass in the study participants.

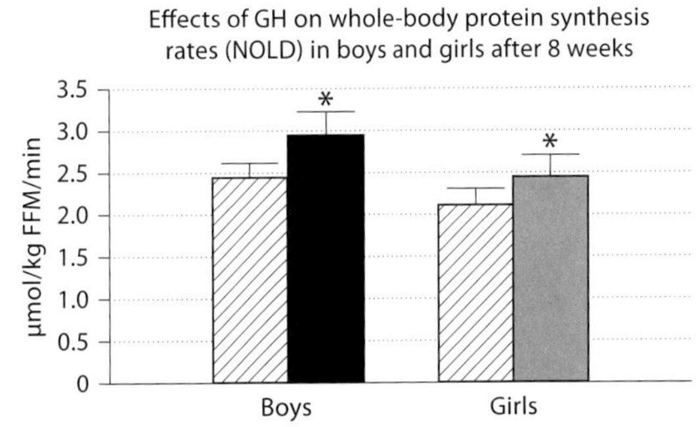

Fig. 1. Changes in nonoxidative leucine disposal (NOLD), a measure of whole-body protein synthesis, in a group of adolescent boys (n = 8) and girls (n = 8) treated for 8 weeks with growth hormone (GH). * $p < 0.05$ vs. baseline (data from Mauras et al. [12]). FFM = Fat-free mass.

Table 1. Metabolic effects of long-term GCs vs. GH/IGF-I

Effect	GCs	GH/GF-I
Leucine oxidation	↑	↓
Whole-body protein and muscle synthesis	↓	↑
Intra-abdominal adiposity	↑	↓
Lean body mass	↓	↑
Muscle atrophy	↑	↓
Insulin sensitivity	↓	↓↑
Bone resorption/osteoporosis	↑	↓←→
Linear growth	↓	↑

GCs = Glucocorticosteroids; GH/IGF-I = growth hormone/insulin-like growth factor I.

Metabolic studies in children also show that GH potently stimulates whole-body protein synthesis, increases lean body mass and decreases adiposity, even after only 8 weeks of therapy [12]. In adolescents treated with GH, IGF-I concentrations were higher in females during GH therapy, but the metabolic effects were not different by gender. There was comparable stimulation of whole-body protein synthesis and favorable body composition in both girls and boys [12] (fig. 1). Table 1 summarizes the metabolic effects of chronic GC use versus those of GH and IGF-I therapy.

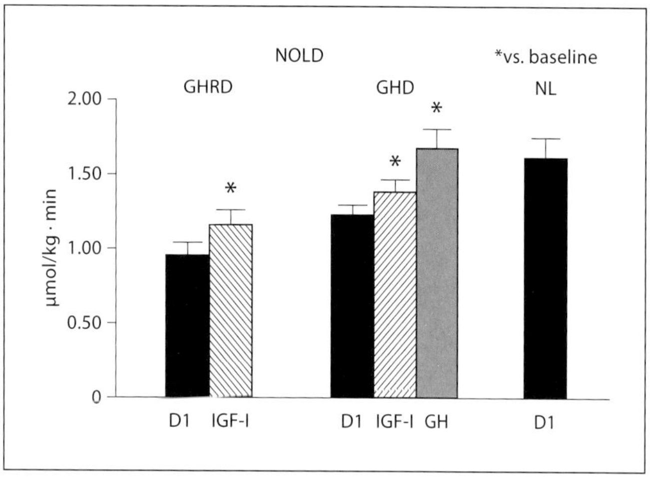

Fig. 2. Comparison of nonoxidative leucine disposal (NOLD), a measure of whole-body protein synthesis, in adults with growth hormone receptor deficiency (GHRD) before and after 8 weeks of IGF-I treatment (n = 10), in adults with GH deficiency (GHD) before and after 8 weeks each of IGF-I and GH treatment (n = 8) and in normal controls (NL; n = 10). The within-group comparisons versus baseline are: GHRD, p = 0.001; GHD after IGF-I, p = 0.06, and GHD after GH, p = 0.02. D1 = Day 1. (Reprinted from Mauras et al. [15] with permission from The Endocrine Society. © 2000, The Endocrine Society.)

In situations of relative caloric deprivation, coadministration of GH and IGF-I appears to be synergistic in enhancing a more positive protein balance [13]; however, in normally fed individuals, the combination does not convey greater protein-anabolic effects than either compound alone [14]. In aggregate, the available data suggest that IGF-I mediates the protein-anabolic actions of GH in humans.

We have also compared the effects of 8 weeks of GH and IGF-I treatment in GH-deficient subjects with those of IGF-I treatment alone in GHR-deficient individuals (Laron syndrome). Compared with control subjects, GH was more effective at normalizing rates of whole-body protein synthesis [15]. IGF-I was also effective in enhancing whole-body protein synthesis in both groups. These findings strongly support the potent protein-anabolic role of these hormones (fig. 2). They also suggest that, similar to GH replacement in GH-deficient adults, IGF-I may be beneficial as a long-term replacement therapy in GHR-deficient individuals for purposes other than growth.

Effects on Carbohydrate Metabolism

Chronic administration of GH results in compensatory hyperinsulinemia and is associated with the development of relative insulin resistance. However, these findings are not typically associated with clinically significant disease; further, most patients receiving GH do not exhibit carbohydrate intolerance [16]. GH replacement therapy in GH-deficient adults results in decreased carbohydrate oxidation rates, as measured by indirect calorimetry, and increased glucose production rates, as measured by stable isotope methods. Both of these findings are most likely secondary to increased insulin resistance [11]. Neither typically results in any change in glucose tolerance. On the other hand, IGF-I administration results in improved insulin sensitivity [10], an observation that has led to the study of IGF-I as a potential adjunct treatment for patients with diabetes [17]. Long-term trials with IGF-I are needed to define better its effect on carbohydrate metabolism in selected populations.

Effects on Fat Metabolism

GH receptors are expressed in the human adipocyte and GH has significant effects on fat metabolism [18]. The positive effects on lipid profiles and deceased adiposity observed after GH replacement therapy are major benefits associated with such therapy in adults [19, 20]. GH replacement therapy is also associated with an improved lipolytic response of isolated adipocytes to epinephrine via increased efficiency of the β-adrenergic pathway and greater receptor numbers [21, 22]. This increased sensitivity to the lipolytic effect of catecholamines is also observed in cultured adipocytes from healthy adults treated with GH [23]. The beneficial lipid profile observed after GH therapy, i.e., decreased total cholesterol, low-density lipoprotein (LDL) cholesterol and Apo B100 (the main protein content of LDL), is probably related in part to the induction of hepatic LDL receptors [24].

There is a substantial redistribution of body fat following GH therapy in children with hypopituitarism. The classic 'pudgy' appearance of the hypopituitary child changes after GH; adiposity decreases and at times the physique remarkably 'thins out' [25]. Utilizing gluteal and abdominal subcutaneous tissue from children treated with GH for 3 months, Rosenbaum et al. found a marked decrease in abdominal adipocyte size, a reduced rate of lipogenesis and variable desensitization of the abdominal depots to the antilipolytic effects of insulin [26]. These effects have also been observed in obese children with Prader-Willi syndrome treated with GH [27]. GH administration, however, typically does not cause weight loss, but rather a change in body composition by increasing fat mobilization, oxidation and protein synthesis and decreasing protein oxidation [11].

Conversely, IGF-I does not mediate the effects of GH on lipids or lipolysis; in addition, there are no functional type 1 IGF-I receptors in adipocytes [18]. However, IGF-I therapy can potently affect lipolysis. We observed substantial changes in body composition, with decreased adiposity and increased lean body mass, lipolysis and lipid oxidation rates, in a unique group of patients with GHR deficiency treated with IGF-I for 8 weeks [15]. However, in a group of healthy postmenopausal women, 1 year of treatment with IGF-I was not associated with any measurable increase in lean body mass or decrease in adiposity [28]. It is possible that the potent effects we observed in patients with Laron syndrome treated with IGF-I were a reflection of the severity and congenital nature of their deficiency and could not be replicated in normal, albeit elderly, subjects. Similarly, GH-deficient patients are more likely to show benefit from long-term GH replacement than normal elderly subjects [19]. Whether long-term IGF-I therapy will result in sustained changes in adiposity requires further study.

GCs and the GH Axis

Several lines of evidence suggest that GCs can negatively affect both GH secretion and GH action at many levels. GCs can impair the release of GH via attenuation of GH transcription in response to GH-releasing hormone (GHRH); even in acute doses, GCs markedly decrease the GH response to GHRH [29, 30]. GCs also decrease hepatic GH receptor expression and hence the generation of IGF-I [31]. At the level of the epiphyseal growth plate, GCs affect local GH receptor expression, IGF-I generation and interactions of IGF-I with its receptor [32, 33]. Therefore, in practical terms, chronic use of steroids results in a state of 'functional' GH deficiency.

Given that GH and IGF-I are substantially anabolic in vivo, can these compounds diminish the catabolic effects of steroids? In classic metabolism studies, Horber and Haymond gave high doses of steroids for 7 days to healthy volunteers to mimic the catabolic state of chronic steroid use [34]. Using stable and radioactive tracers of the essential amino acid leucine, they demonstrated that GH abolished the protein-wasting effects of steroids in humans. However, steroids and GH each caused significant insulin resistance, which appeared to be additive when GH and steroids were used together [35]. Using IGF-I in GC-treated subjects, we observed similar protein-anabolic effects [36]. However, contrary to GH, IGF-I treatment in these subjects was associated with normal glucose concentrations despite marked reductions in circulating insulin, indicative of the potent insulin-like activity of the peptide [36]. This offers an important theoretical advantage over GH when considering long-term treatment of a steroid-treated patient; however, this issue is yet to be properly studied. Nevertheless, these data underscore the importance of careful monitoring of carbohydrate tolerance in patients treated with steroids and GH.

In rats treated with either GCs or GH, GCs decreased growth and modeling of the bone, while GH increased the cortical bone mass, but not the mineralizing surface of cancellous bone [37, 38]. These data suggest that GH may decrease, at least in part, the negative effects of steroids on bone. Collectively, these and other data support the concept that both GH and IGF-I may play a role in ameliorating the catabolic effects of steroids.

Overview of Catabolic States Sensitive to GH

Steroid-Dependent Inflammatory Bowel Disease

In a 4-month pilot trial, ten children with profound growth retardation secondary to inflammatory bowel disease and chronic steroid use were treated with GH [39]. We observed significant improvement in linear growth, decreased adiposity and improved lean body mass (fig. 3). We also showed increases in measures of bone calcium accretion (using stable isotopes of calcium) and in markers of bone formation. There were no substantial differences in fasting or 2-hour postprandial glucose concentrations, glycosylated hemoglobin or measures of hepatic glucose production after 4 months of treatment.

Cystic Fibrosis

Cystic fibrosis is another condition of chronic inflammation and often severe catabolism in which children may grow very poorly, with or without concomitant treatment with steroids [40]. We have studied children with cystic fibrosis using stable isotopic infusions of amino acids during treatment with GH alone, glutamine (a nonessential amino acid) alone and GH plus glutamine [41]. Oral glutamine did not promote protein gain in the fasting state, while a short course of GH had a potent anabolic effect that is mediated by stimulation of protein synthesis without affecting glutamine kinetics [41]. In a multicenter, randomized, controlled trial using GH in this patient population, Hardin et al. also showed that GH improves growth and clinical status [42]. Collectively, the data suggest a potent effect of GH on the catabolic state

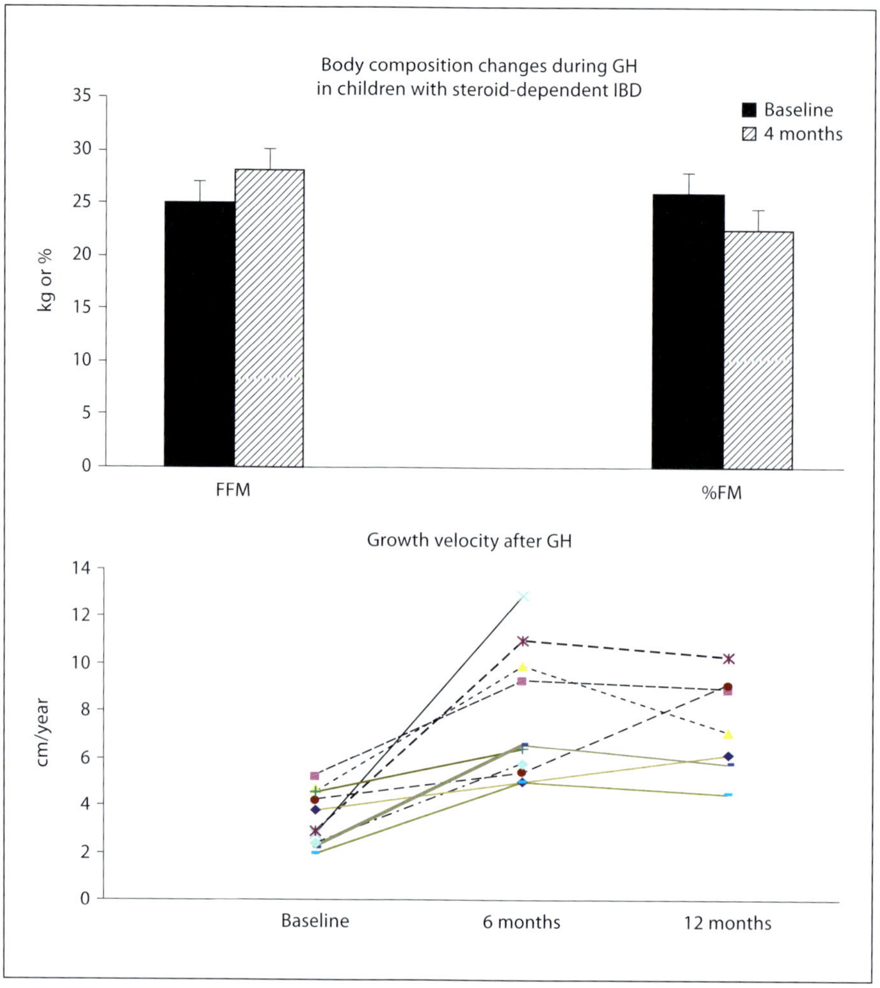

Fig. 3. Top: body composition analysis by dual-energy X-ray absorptiometry performed at baseline and 4 months after growth hormone (GH) treatment in prednisone-dependent children with inflammatory bowel disease (IBD; n = 10). Changes in fat-free mass (FFM) (+3 kg) and percent fat mass (%FM) (–3.5%) were significant (p = 0.001) after treatment. Bottom: growth velocity of the same subjects at baseline and after 6 months of continuous GH therapy. Seven patients continued treatment for 12 months. (Reprinted from Mauras et al. [39] with permission from Elsevier. © 2002, Elsevier.)

in children with cystic fibrosis, many of whom are also treated with steroids.

Juvenile Idiopathic Arthritis

Juvenile idiopathic arthritis (JIA) is a further critical example of the potential role of GH in antagonizing the catabolic effects of the underlying inflammatory process, as well as the effects of long-term steroid therapy, on growth. Simon et al. treated children with JIA and steroid dependency in a randomized trial using either GH or no GH for 3 years [43]. Mean height standard deviation score (SDS) increase was greater in patients receiving GH (0.37 ± 1.5 SDS) than in patients not receiving GH (–0.96 ± 1.2 SDS) (p = 0.04). Mean height velocity returned to normal within the first year of GH treatment and remained normal thereafter, and the increase in mean lean body mass was greater in GH-treated patients (7.3 ± 2.9 vs. 4.4 ± 2.8 kg; p = 0.03). Fat mass and bone mineralization were not significantly different in the two groups. Fasting serum insulin increased significantly in GH-treated patients (5.2 ± 16 mIU/l) compared with untreated patients (–2.3 ± 5 mIU/l) (p = 0.04), and fasting glycemia was unchanged. The authors concluded that, when started early in the course of JIA, GH therapy preserved normal growth velocity and height. Although GH was well tolerated, carbohydrate metabolism should be monitored closely.

Summary and Conclusions

With chronic use, GCs can cause a severe catabolic imbalance. Many of the catabolic and growth-suppressive effects of GCs are mediated via interference in translational mechanisms in the GH/IGF-I axis and by diminishing GH secretion. Hence, chronic steroid use creates a state of functional GH deficiency. In vitro and in vivo data on catabolic states suggest that therapy with GH and possibly IGF-I, which are potent anabolic hormones, may diminish or abolish the protein-catabolic and growth-suppressive effects of chronic steroid use and chronic inflammation. However, the combination of chronic inflammation, chronic steroid use and GH therapy produces insulin resistance and compensatory hyperinsulinemia. Therefore, careful monitoring of carbohydrate metabolism in patients who have chronic illnesses or require chronic steroid use is critical, especially when GH replacement therapy is administered. GH and possibly IGF-I offer promise in the treatment of growth disorders in children with catabolic conditions, although further longitudinal studies are needed to better judge the safety and efficacy of this approach.

Disclosure Statement

The author has acted as a consultant for Tercica and has received honoraria from Pfizer.

References

1 Schakman O, Gilson H, Thissen JP: Mechanisms of glucocorticoid-induced myopathy. J Endocrinol 2008;197:1–10.
2 Beaufrere B, Horber FF, Schwenk WF, Marsh HM, Matthews D, Gerich JE, Haymond MW: Glucocorticosteroids increase leucine oxidation and impair leucine balance in humans. Am J Physiol 1989;257:E712–E721.
3 Mayo-Smith W, Hayes CW, Biller BMK, Klibanski A, Rosenthal H, Rosenthal DI: Body fat distribution measured with CT: correlations in healthy subjects, patients with anorexia nervosa, and patients with Cushing syndrome. Radiology 1989;170: 515–518.
4 Rosenfeld R, Reiter EO: Normal and aberrant growth; in Kronenberg HM, Melmed S, Polonsky KS, Larsen PR (eds): Williams Textbook of Endocrinology, 2008, ed 11. Philadelphia, Saunders, pp 849–968.
5 Greenhalgh CJ, Alexander WS: Suppressors of cytokine signalling and regulation of growth hormone action. Growth Horm IGF Res 2004;14:200–206.
6 Metcalf D, Greenhalgh CJ, Viney E, Willson TA, Starr R, Nicola NA, Hilton DJ, Alexander WS: Gigantism in mice lacking suppressor of cytokine signalling-2. Nature 2000; 405:1069–1073.
7 Rinderknecht E, Humbel RE: The amino acid sequence of human insulin-like growth factor I and its structural homology with proinsulin. J Biol Chem 1978;253:2769–2776.
8 Werner H, Woloschak M, Stannard B, Shen-Orr A, Roberts CT Jr, LeRoith D: The insulin-like growth factor I receptor: molecular biology, heterogeneity, and regulation; in LeRoith D (ed): Insulin-Like Growth Factors: Molecular and Cellular Aspects. Boca Raton, CRC Press, 1991, pp 17–47.
9 Di Cola G, Cool MH, Accili D: Hypoglycemic effect of insulin-like growth factor-1 in mice lacking insulin receptors. J Clin Invest 1997;99:2538–2544.
10 Mauras N, Haymond MW: Are the metabolic effects of GH and IGF-I separable? Growth Horm IGF Res 2005;15:19–27.
11 Mauras N, O'Brien KO, Welch S, Rini A, Helgeson K, Vieira NE, Yergey AL: Insulin-like growth factor I and growth hormone (GH) treatment in GH-deficient humans: differential effects on protein, glucose, lipid and calcium metabolism. J Clin Endocrinol Metab 2000;85:1686–1694.
12 Mauras N, Bishop K, Welch S: Growth hormone action in puberty: effects by gender. Growth Horm IGF Res 2007;17:463–471.
13 Kupfer SR, Underwood LE, Baxter RC, Clemmons DR: Enhancement of the anabolic effects of growth hormone and insulin-like growth factor I by use of both agents simultaneously. J Clin Invest 1993;91:391–396.
14 Mauras N: Combined recombinant human growth hormone and recombinant human insulin-like growth factor I: lack of synergy on whole body protein anabolism in normally fed subjects. J Clin Endocrinol Metab 1995;80:2633–2637.
15 Mauras N, Martinez V, Rini A, Guevara-Aguirre J: Recombinant human insulin-like growth factor I has significant anabolic effects in adults with growth hormone receptor deficiency: studies on protein, glucose, and lipid metabolism. J Clin Endocrinol Metab 2000;85:3036–3042.
16 Saenger P, Attie KM, Dimartino-Nardi J, Hintz R, Frahm L, Frane JW: Metabolic consequences of 5-year growth hormone (GH) therapy in children treated with GH for idiopathic short stature. Genentech Collaborative Study Group. J Clin Endocrinol Metab 1998;83:3115–3120.
17 Acerini CL, Patton CM, Savage MO, Kernell A, Westphal O, Dunger DB: Randomised placebo-controlled trial of human recombinant insulin-like growth factor I plus intensive insulin therapy in adolescents with insulin-dependent diabetes mellitus. Lancet 1997;350:1199–1204.
18 DiGirolamo M, Edén S, Enberg G, Isaksson O, Lönnroth P, Hall K, Smith U: Specific binding of human growth hormone but not insulin-like growth factors by human adipocytes. FEBS Lett 1986;205:15–19.
19 Vance ML, Mauras N: Growth hormone therapy in adults and children. N Engl J Med 1999;341:1206–1216.
20 Carroll PV, Christ ER, Bengtsson BA, Carlsson L, Christiansen JS, Clemmons D, Hintz R, Ho K, Laron Z, Sizonenko P, Sönksen PH, Tanaka T, Thorne M: Growth hormone deficiency in adulthood and the effects of growth hormone replacement: a review. Growth Hormone Research Society Scientific Committee. J Clin Endocrinol Metab 1998;83: 382–395.
21 Beauville M, Harant I, Crampes F, Riviere D, Tauber MT, Tauber JP, Garrigues M: Effect of long-term rhGH administration in GH-deficient adults on fat cell epinephrine response. Am J Physiol 1992;263:E467–E472.
22 Yang S, Björntorp P, Liu X, Edén S: Growth hormone treatment of hypophysectomized rats increases catecholamine-induced lipolysis and the number of β-adrenergic receptors in adipocytes: no differences in the effects of GH on different fat depots. Obes Res 1996;4:471–478.
23 Marcus C, Bolme P, Micha-Johansson G, Margery V, Brönnegård M: Growth hormone increases the lipolytic sensitivity for catecholamines in adipocytes from healthy adults. Life Sci 1994;54:1335–1341.
24 Rudling M, Norstedt G, Olivecrona H, Reihner E, Gustafsson JA, Angelin B: Importance of growth hormone for the induction of hepatic low density lipoprotein receptors. Proc Natl Acad Sci USA 1992;89:6983–6987.
25 Mauras N: Metabolic effects of insulin-like growth factor I and growth hormone in vivo: a comparison; in Le Roith D, Zumkeller W, Baxter RC (eds): Insulin-Like Growth Factor Receptor Signalling. New York, Kluwer Academic Plenum Publishers, 2003, pp 423–433.

26 Rosenbaum M, Gertner JM, Leibel RL: Effects of systemic growth hormone (GH) administration on regional adipose tissue distribution and metabolism in GH-deficient children. J Clin Endocrinol Metab 1989;69: 1274–1281.
27 Myers SE, Carrel AL, Whitman BY, Allen DB: Sustained benefit after 2 years of growth hormone on body composition, fat utilization, physical strength and agility, and growth in Prader-Willi syndrome. J Pediatr 2000;137:42–49.
28 Friedlander AL, Butterfield GE, Moynihan S, Grillo J, Pollack M, Holloway L, Friedman L, Yesavage J, Matthias D, Lee S, Marcus R, Hoffman AR: One year of insulin-like growth factor I treatment does not affect bone density, body composition, or psychological measures in postmenopausal women. J Clin Endocrinol Metab 2001;86:1496–1503.
29 Kaufmann S, Jones KL, Wehrenberg WB, Culler FL: Inhibition by prednisone of growth hormone (GH) response to GH-releasing hormone in normal men. J Clin Endocrinol Metab 1988;67:1258–1261.
30 Miell JP, Corder R, Pralong FP, Gaillard RC: Effects of dexamethasone on growth hormone (GH)-releasing hormone, arginine- and dopaminergic stimulated GH secretion, and total plasma insulin-like growth factor-I concentrations in normal male volunteers. J Clin Endocrinol Metab 1991;72:675–681.
31 Kritsch KR, Murali S, Adamo ML, Ney DM: Dexamethasone decreases serum and liver IGF-I and maintains liver IGF-I mRNA in parenterally fed rats. Am J Physiol Regul Integr Comp Physiol 2002;282:R528–R536.
32 Smink JJ, Gresnigt MG, Hamers N, Koedam JA, Berger R, Van Buul-Offers SC: Short-term glucocorticoid treatment of prepubertal mice decreases growth and IGF-I expression in the growth plate. J Endocrinol 2003; 177:381–388.
33 Mehls O, Himmele R, Hömme M, Kiepe D, Klaus G: The interaction of glucocorticoids with the growth hormone-insulin-like growth factor axis and its effects on growth plate chondrocytes and bone cells. J Pediatr Endocrinol Metab 2001;14(suppl 6):1475–1482.
34 Horber FF, Haymond MW: Human growth hormone prevents the protein catabolic side effects of prednisone in humans. J Clin Invest 1990;86:265–272.
35 Horber FF, Marsh HM, Haymond MW: Differential effects of prednisone and growth hormone on fuel metabolism and insulin antagonism in humans. Diabetes 1991;40:141–149.
36 Mauras N, Beaufrere B: Recombinant human insulin-like growth factor-I enhances whole body protein anabolism and significantly diminishes the protein catabolic effects of prednisone in humans without a diabetogenic effect. J Clin Endocrinol Metab 1995;80:869–874.
37 Ortoft G, Andreassen TT, Oxlund H: Growth hormone increases cortical and cancellous bone mass in young growing rats with glucocorticoid-induced osteopenia. J Bone Miner Res 1999;14:710–721.
38 Ortoft G, Andreassen TT, Oxlund H: Growth hormone can reverse glucocorticoid-induced low bone turnover on cortical but not on cancellous bone surfaces in adult Wistar rats. Bone 2005;36:123–133.
39 Mauras N, George D, Evans J, Milov D, Abrams S, Rini A, Welch S, Haymond MW: Growth hormone has anabolic effects in glucocorticosteroid-dependent children with inflammatory bowel disease: a pilot study. Metabolism 2002;51:127–135.
40 Lai HC, FitzSimmons SC, Allen DB, Kosorok MR, Rosenstein BJ, Campbell PW, Farrell PM: Risk of persistent growth impairment after alternate-day prednisone treatment in children with cystic fibrosis. N Engl J Med 2000;342:851–859.
41 Darmaun D, Hayes V, Schaeffer D, Welch S, Mauras N: Effects of glutamine and recombinant human growth hormone on protein metabolism in prepubertal children with cystic fibrosis. J Clin Endocrinol Metab 2004;89:1146–1152.
42 Hardin DS, Adams-Huet B, Brown D, Chatfield B, Dyson M, Ferkol T, Howenstine M, Prestidge C, Royce F, Rice J, Seilheimer DK, Steelman J, Shepherds R: Growth hormone treatment improves growth and clinical status in prepubertal children with cystic fibrosis: results of a multicenter randomized controlled trial. J Clin Endocrinol Metab 2006; 91:4925–4929.
43 Simon D, Prieur AM, Quartier P, Charles Ruiz J, Czernichow P: Early recombinant human growth hormone treatment in glucocorticoid-treated children with juvenile idiopathic arthritis: a 3-year randomized study. J Clin Endocrinol Metab 2007;92: 2567–2573.

HORMONE RESEARCH

Horm Res 2009;72(suppl 1):55–59
DOI: 10.1159/000229765

Published online: November 27, 2009

Effects of Growth Hormone Treatment on Growth in Children with Juvenile Idiopathic Arthritis

D. Simon[a] S. Bechtold[b]

[a]Department of Endocrinology and Diabetology, Hôpital Robert Debré, Paris, France;
[b]Division of Pediatric Endocrinology, University Children's Hospital, Munich, Germany

Key Words

Juvenile idiopathic arthritis · Growth hormone · Growth retardation · Glucocorticoids

Abstract

Background: Several therapeutic trials have been conducted over the past decade to evaluate the role of exogenous growth hormone (GH) as a means of correcting the growth deficiency seen in children with juvenile idiopathic arthritis (JIA). Early studies showed the benefit of GH treatment with respect to final height in patients with JIA. Of 13 patients receiving GH, 84% (11 patients) achieved a final height within their target range compared with only 22% (4 of 18 patients) of untreated patients. There are, however, factors that may limit the statural gains achieved with GH therapy including severe inflammation, severe statural deficiency at GH therapy initiation, long disease duration and delayed puberty. Data on the efficacy of GH replacement therapy in children with JIA and factors that influence the statural growth response will be reviewed. ***Conclusions:*** Results from therapeutic trials show that treatment with GH can decrease the statural deficit that occurs during the active phase of JIA, producing an adult height that is close to the genetically determined target height.

Introduction

Growth deficiency is a common complication of juvenile idiopathic arthritis (JIA). There is an early decrease in linear growth that correlates with disease severity, and 'catch-up' growth does not occur consistently after disease remission. Final height is less than –2 standard deviations (SDs) in 11% of patients with polyarticular JIA [1] and in 40% of those with systemic JIA [2]. Studies have found both normal and diminished plasma growth hormone (GH) levels, with low plasma insulin-like growth factor-I (IGF-I) levels in some patients [3, 4]. Inflammation and glucocorticoid treatment may induce insensitivity to GH [5]. Because GH stimulates growth, protein anabolism, lipolysis and bone mineralization, several trials have been conducted to determine whether GH replacement therapy is effective in counteracting the deleterious effects of chronic inflammation and glucocorticoid therapy. The short- and long-term effects of GH therapy in patients with JIA and the factors that influence the growth response to GH will be reviewed.

Trials of GH Therapy: Effects on Growth

Short- and Medium-Term Results

The first clinical studies designed to assess the effects of GH therapy on growth in children with JIA focused on

KARGER

Fax +41 61 306 12 34
E-Mail karger@karger.ch
www.karger.com

0301–0163/09/0727–0055 $26.00/0

Accessible online at:
www.karger.com/hre

Dr. Dominique Simon
Department of Endocrinology and Diabetology, Hôpital Robert Debré
48, boulevard Sérurier, FR–75019 Paris (France)
Tel. +33 1 40 03 3634, Fax +33 1 40 03 2429
E-Mail dominique.simon@rdb.aphp.fr

Table 1. Published studies of short- and medium-term (1–4 years) effects of growth hormone (GH) therapy on growth velocity (GV) and height (in SD) of glucocorticoid-treated patients with juvenile idiopathic arthritis

Author (year) [Ref.]	Study type	Pa-tients	Age at start of GH years	GH dose mg/kg/wk	Duration of GH treatment years	GV at baseline cm/year	GV year 1 year 2 year 3 year 4	Height SDS at baseline	Height year 1 year 2 year 3 year 4	Prednisone dose	Disease dura-tion years
Butenandt (1979) [6]	Observational	20	13.0	0.1–0.2	1–2	2.7	6.2 (n = 12) (year 1)	NA	NA	0.17 mg/kg/d	8.2
Svantesson (1991) [7]	Observational	6	13.7	0.16–0.46	0.5–3	2.8	6.7 (year 1)	–3.4	NA	≤5 mg/d	9.2
Davies et al. (1994) [8]	Observational	10 10	9.2 10.6	0.15 0.3	1	2.4 2.0	4.5 (year 1) 6.1 (year 1)	–3.0 –3.4	NA	5–11 mg/d	6.2 7.0
Touati et al. (1998) [9]	Observational	15	9.8	0.46	1	1.9	5.4 (year 1)	–4.3	–4.3 (year 1)	0.38 mg/kg/d	6.5
Simon et al. (2003) [10]	Observational	13	12.4	0.46	3	2.1	6.0 (year 1) 5.0 (year 2) 4.1 (year 3)	–4.6	–4.5 (year 1) –4.5 (year 2) –4.3 (year 3)	0.39 mg/kg/d	8.2
Bechtold et al. (2003) [11]	Controlled	18 T 20 C	10.1	0.2–0.33	4	2.4 2.3	4.7 (year 4) 3.4 (year 4)	–3.3 –2.3	–2.3 (year 4) –3.0 (year 4)	0.2 mg/kg/d 0.2 mg/kg/d	6.3

NA = Not applicable; SDS = standard deviation score; T = treated; C = control.

patients with polyarticular or systemic forms of the disease with several years' duration, glucocorticoid dependency and severe growth deficiency (table 1) [6–11]. GH dosages ranged from 0.1 to 0.46 mg/kg/week. GH replacement therapy markedly increased linear growth velocity, which returned to normal within the first treatment year. This acceleration in linear growth was associated with significant increases in serum levels of IGF-I and IGF-binding protein-3 (IGFBP-3), which persisted as long as GH therapy was continued [9] and indicated a preserved sensitivity to GH. However, in contrast to data obtained with GH use in other indications, catch-up growth did not occur consistently; there is marked interindividual variability [12]. Continued GH replacement for up to 3 years halted the statural loss usually seen during the active phase of JIA and kept patients on the growth curve that corresponded to their height at treatment initiation [10]. In a randomized controlled trial of GH therapy in 31 children with JIA, patients receiving GH (0.33 mg/kg/week for 4 years) had an increase in height of 1 SD compared with a decrease of 0.7 SD in the untreated control group [11].

Long-Term Results: Final Height

Long-term data from the above-mentioned randomized, controlled trial indicated that final height was achieved after a mean follow-up of 7 years [13] (fig. 1). Mean final height (± SD) was significantly greater in the GH-treated patients (–1.6 ± 0.25) compared with control patients (–3.4 ± 2.0); $p < 0.001$. The treated patients had a mean height gain of 1.6 ± 0.8 SD compared with a mean height loss of 0.7 ± 1.8 SD in nontreated patients during the same period. GH therapy did not affect age at puberty (13 years in both groups). Height gain in the treated patients was greater during puberty (21.0 ± 7.3 cm, +1.04 ± 1.1 SD over 5.3 years) than before puberty (17.0 ± 6.5 cm, 0.53 ± 0.8 SD over 2.8 years) and was significantly greater than in control patients (before puberty, 10.5 ± 6.2 cm, –0.85 ± 1.7 SD over 3.4 years; during puberty, 13.3 ± 7.5 cm, 0.12 ± 0.9 SD over 5 years).

Factors That Influence the Growth Response to GH Therapy

Studies in patients with JIA consistently show considerable variability in the linear growth response to GH therapy. Further, they have identified several factors that influence spontaneous growth and GH-induced growth in the short and long term. Severe inflammation is associated with insensitivity to GH and therefore substantial-

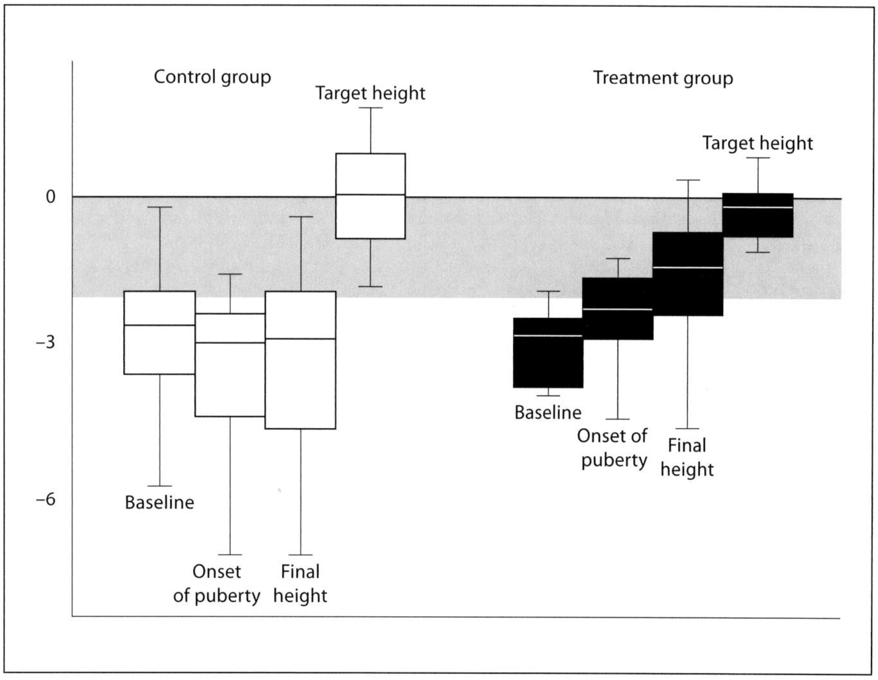

Fig. 1. Height changes (in standard deviation) in two groups of children with juvenile idiopathic arthritis, one treated with growth hormone (0.33 mg/kg/week) (right) and the other an untreated control group (left). Height is given at study inclusion, at the start of puberty and at final height, with the genetically determined target height for comparison. (Reprinted from Bechtold et al. [13] with permission from The Endocrine Society. © 2007, The Endocrine Society.)

ly decreases the short- and long-term efficacy of GH therapy. Thus, patients with polyarticular disease gain more height with GH therapy than do patients with systemic disease [9]. Similarly, the height gain seen with GH therapy correlates negatively with inflammation severity as assessed by laboratory markers (erythrocyte sedimentation rate or C-reactive protein) and/or with glucocorticoid dosing during GH therapy. Laboratory markers of inflammation are also associated with the long-term linear growth response and final height of patients with JIA [13].

The GH dosage across trials ranged from 0.1 to 0.33 mg/kg/week; however, higher dosages of up to 0.46 mg/kg/week have been used in patients with JIA. The rationale for using higher dosages of GH is that chronic inflammation and glucocorticoid therapy decrease the sensitivity to GH. The short-term response to GH therapy showed a dose-response effect with higher GH dosages associated with greater height gains after 1 year [8, 11]. However, no published studies have compared the effects of various GH dosages on the final height of patients with JIA. The positive correlation between final height and mean plasma levels of IGF-I and IGFBP-3 during GH therapy suggests an influence of GH dosage on long-term height gain.

When Should GH Therapy Be Started?

GH replacement therapy in JIA was first evaluated in patients who had severe growth deficiency after several years of glucocorticoid therapy, and the results on final height were promising. Although age at GH therapy initiation and duration of GH therapy have not been directly evaluated with regards to effect on final height, several clinical and experimental arguments support early GH therapy. First, the course of JIA is unpredictable, and some patients experience inflammatory flare-ups that limit the efficacy of GH therapy. Second, experimental studies show that the duration of cytokine and glucocorticoid exposure influences the severity of growth plate damage [14–17] and may affect the potential for spontaneous or GH-induced catch-up growth. Finally, height at puberty correlates with final height in both GH-treated and untreated patients, suggesting that earlier GH therapy to achieve catch-up growth before puberty onset may result in greater final height. A recently published randomized trial in children with JIA investigated the effects of high-dose GH therapy (0.46 mg/kg/week) started early – within 12–15 months after glucocorticoid therapy initiation – at a time when height was still normal [18]. The results were encouraging. The heights of GH-treated children remained normal throughout the 3 years of follow-up (–1.1 SD at baseline and –0.3 SD after 3 years). In

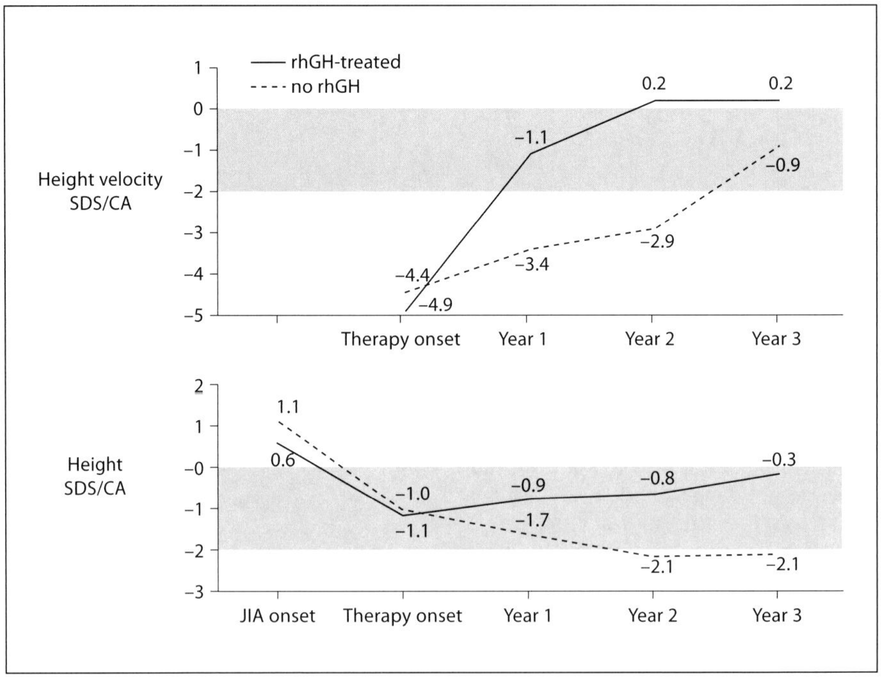

Fig. 2. Changes over 3 years in growth velocity (top) and height (bottom) in standard deviation score/chronological age (SDS/CA) in patients with juvenile idiopathic arthritis with (solid lines) and without (dashed lines) growth hormone therapy started within 1 year after glucocorticoid therapy initiation. (Reprinted from Simon et al. [18] with permission from The Endocrine Society. © 2007, The Endocrine Society.)

contrast, during the same period, the control patients experienced slowing of linear growth with a height decrease from –1.0 SD to –2.1 SD (fig. 2). Over the 3-year study period, the GH-treated patients experienced a mean height gain of 0.37 ± 1.5 SD compared with a mean height loss of 0.96 ± 1.2 SD in control patients. Thus, early GH therapy was effective in preventing growth deficiency and in maintaining normal height over the first 3 years of the disease. Long-term data from these patients will determine whether early high-dose GH therapy improves final height and body composition.

Who Should Be Offered GH Therapy?

Growth monitoring is an important part of the follow-up of children with chronic inflammatory diseases. Pediatric rheumatologists must ensure that growth disturbances are detected and treated early. Factors associated with a high risk of growth deficiency are early onset of disease, severe and prolonged inflammation (polyarticular and systemic forms of JIA) and severe glucocorticoid dependency. Available data suggest that initiation of GH therapy may be appropriate as soon as growth deficiency is detected (i.e., height ≤–2 SD). In patients seen late in the course of their disease with severe growth deficiency and delayed puberty, GH therapy may provide some measure of catch-up growth during puberty. In patients with delayed puberty, combining GH therapy with sex steroid therapy may optimize the height gain and improve body composition (by increasing fat-free mass and bone mass). However, no published data showing benefits from this combination are available to date.

Conclusions

We now have findings from more than two decades of clinical studies in children with JIA. Results show that GH therapy improves linear growth during the active phase of the disease, thereby increasing final height. Over the next few years, studies in larger patient populations designed to identify factors that influence the growth response to GH will help to 'fine-tune' GH therapy. In particular, the optimal time for treatment initiation and the optimal dose need to be determined. Whether combined sex steroid and GH therapy optimizes the growth response in patients with delayed puberty requires additional evaluation.

Disclosure Statement

D.S. has received honoraria from Pfizer. S.B. declares no conflict of interest.

References

1 Zak M, Muller J, Karup Pedersen F: Final height, armspan, subischial leg length and body proportions in juvenile chronic arthritis. A long-term follow-up study. Horm Res 1999;52:80–85.

2 Simon D, Fernando C, Czernichow P, Prieur AM: Linear growth and final height in patients with systemic juvenile idiopathic arthritis treated with longterm glucocorticoids. J Rheumatol 2002;29:1296–1300.

3 Allen RC, Jimenez M, Cowell CT: Insulin-like growth factor and growth hormone secretion in juvenile chronic arthritis. Ann Rheum Dis 1991;50:602–606.

4 Bennett AE, Silverman ED, Miller JJ 3rd, Hintz RL: Insulin-like growth factors i and ii in children with systemic onset juvenile arthritis. J Rheumatol 1988;15:655–658.

5 Bergad PL, Schwarzenberg SJ, Humbert JT, Morrison M, Amarasinghe S, Towle HC, Berry SA: Inhibition of growth hormone action in models of inflammation. Am J Physiol Cell Physiol 2000;279:C1906–C1917.

6 Butenandt O: Rheumatoid arthritis and growth retardation in children: treatment with human growth hormone. Eur J Pediatr 1979;130:15–28.

7 Svantesson H: Treatment of growth failure with human growth hormone in patients with juvenile chronic arthritis. A pilot study. Clin Exp Rheumatol 1991;9(suppl 6):47–50.

8 Davies UM, Rooney M, Preece MA, Ansell BM, Woo P: Treatment of growth retardation in juvenile chronic arthritis with recombinant human growth hormone. J Rheumatol 1994;21:153–158.

9 Touati G, Prieur AM, Ruiz JC, Noel M, Czernichow P: Beneficial effects of one-year growth hormone administration to children with juvenile chronic arthritis on chronic steroid therapy. I. Effects on growth velocity and body composition. J Clin Endocrinol Metab 1998;83:403–409.

10 Simon D, Lucidarme N, Prieur AM, Ruiz JC, Czernichow P: Effects on growth and body composition of growth hormone treatment in children with juvenile idiopathic arthritis requiring steroid therapy. J Rheumatol 2003; 30:2492–2499.

11 Bechtold S, Ripperger P, Hafner R, Said E, Schwarz HP: Growth hormone improves height in patients with juvenile idiopathic arthritis: 4-year data of a controlled study. J Pediatr 2003;143:512–519.

12 Simon D: rhGH treatment in corticosteroid-treated patients. Horm Res 2007;68:38–45.

13 Bechtold S, Ripperger P, Dalla Pozza R, Bonfig W, Hafner R, Michels H, Schwarz HP: Growth hormone increases final height in patients with juvenile idiopathic arthritis: data from a randomized controlled study. J Clin Endocrinol Metab 2007;92:3013–3018.

14 Jux C, Leiber K, Hugel U, Blum W, Ohlsson C, Klaus G, Mehls O: Dexamethasone impairs growth hormone (GH)-stimulated growth by suppression of local insulin-like growth factor (IGF)-I production and expression of GH- and IGF-I-receptor in cultured rat chondrocytes. Endocrinology 1998; 139:3296–3305.

15 Schrier L, Ferns SP, Barnes KM, Emons JA, Newman EI, Nilsson O, Baron J: Depletion of resting zone chondrocytes during growth plate senescence. J Endocrinol 2006;189:27–36.

16 Mushtaq T, Farquharson C, Seawright E, Ahmed SF: Glucocorticoid effects on chondrogenesis, differentiation and apoptosis in the murine atdc5 chondrocyte cell line. J Endocrinol 2002;175:705–713.

17 MacRae VE, Farquharson C, Ahmed SF: The restricted potential for recovery of growth plate chondrogenesis and longitudinal bone growth following exposure to pro-inflammatory cytokines. J Endocrinol 2006;189: 319–328.

18 Simon D, Prieur AM, Quartier P, Charles Ruiz J, Czernichow P: Early recombinant human growth hormone treatment in glucocorticoid-treated children with juvenile idiopathic arthritis: a 3-year randomized study. J Clin Endocrinol Metab 2007;92: 2567–2573.

HORMONE
RESEARCH

Horm Res 2009;72(suppl 1):60–64
DOI: 10.1159/000229766

Published online: November 27, 2009

Effects of Growth Hormone Treatment in Juvenile Idiopathic Arthritis: Bone and Body Composition

S. Bechtold[a] R. Dalla Pozza[a] H.P. Schwarz[a] D. Simon[b]

[a]Division of Pediatric Endocrinology, University Children's Hospital, Munich, Germany; [b]Department of Endocrinology and Diabetology, Robert Debré Hospital, University of Paris V, Paris, France

Key Words
Juvenile idiopathic arthritis · Growth hormone

Abstract
Background: Inflammation and glucocorticoid therapy are major factors influencing growth and bone maturation in patients with juvenile idiopathic arthritis (JIA). In addition to alterations in total bone mineral density and bone geometry, longitudinal data confirm that the main contributors to errant bone maturation in patients with JIA are reductions in muscle mass and force. Growth hormone (GH) therapy, which has shown efficacy in controlling disease, may also positively influence body composition. For several years, GH therapy has been used to treat growth retardation in patients with JIA receiving glucocorticoids. GH therapy normalizes growth velocity, increases height, bone mineral density and bone mass and changes bone geometry. Despite ongoing glucocorticoid therapy, muscle mass and bone size substantially increase with GH therapy. Increased bone size suggests improved bone stability, which may reduce fracture risk. Along with the increase in muscle mass, patients experience stabilized or slightly decreased fat mass during GH therapy. ***Conclusions:*** All these effects suggest an anabolic effect of GH therapy on bone and body composition.

Introduction

Studies on human bone development have long focused on changes in bone mineral mass (expressed as bone mineral content [BMC]) and bone mineral density (BMD). These indices were initially developed for the diagnosis and follow-up of adults with osteoporosis. Although they can provide useful information about the growing skeleton, interpretation of bone maturation based only on accumulation of mineral mass can be problematic. Bone is a 3-dimensional complex and structural aspects must be considered [1].

Body height is determined by linear growth of bone; however, the width and size of bone also correlate with linear growth. Bone width and size influence bone strength, which is measured by an index of bending resistance. The bending strength of the long bone diaphysis is related to its diameter raised to the third power [2]. Bones are part of the locomotive apparatus and therefore should be analyzed within the context of their mechanical environment. The largest physiological loads on the skeleton result from muscle contraction, not from body weight; therefore, the musculoskeletal system has to be analyzed as a functional unit. Bone strength is usually adequately adapted to local muscle force. If muscle force is low, bone strength is also decreased. Furthermore, it is necessary not only to evaluate the adaptation of bone strength to muscle mass, but also to test whether muscle

KARGER

Fax +41 61 306 12 34
E-Mail karger@karger.ch
www.karger.com

0301–0163/09/0727–0060$26.00/0

Accessible online at:
www.karger.com/hre

Dr. Dominique Simon
Department of Endocrinology and Diabetology, Hôpital Robert Debré
48, boulevard Sérurier, FR–75019 Paris (France)
Tel. +33 1 40 03 3634, Fax +33 1 40 03 2429
E-Mail dominique.simon@rdb.aphp.fr

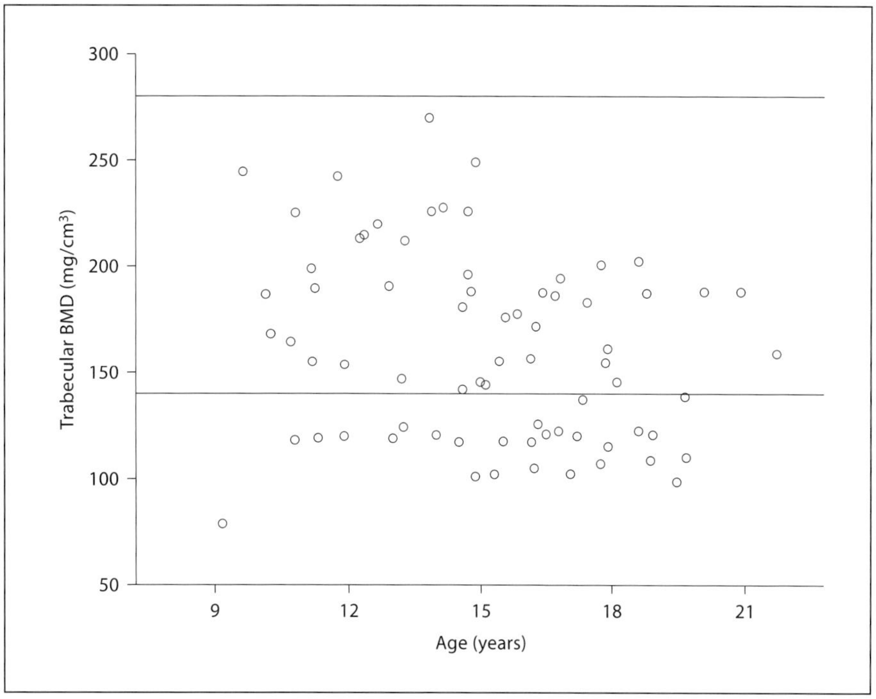

Fig. 1. Longitudinal development of trabecular BMD in patients with juvenile idiopathic arthritis treated with growth hormone in relation to age. Cross bars show the normative range, which is almost constant throughout the life span. BMD = Bone mineral density.

mass or force is normal. Thus, muscle parameters also relate to body height [3].

In children and adolescents with severe forms of juvenile idiopathic arthritis (JIA), growth failure and muscle loss are the most frequently reported extra-articular complications. Other well-recognized findings are reduced BMD and changes in bone geometry. One noteworthy consequence is an increased rate of fragility fractures due to delayed and suboptimal peak bone mass accrual [4]. Low bone mass is not restricted to the very severe end of the disease spectrum or to patients receiving glucocorticoid (GC) treatment. It has also been reported in postpubertal females with JIA who had never received GCs [5].

A number of factors are thought to play a role in the bone loss observed in patients with JIA: the disease activity itself, medication, reduced physical activity and malnutrition. Loss of muscle mass has been described as a central factor for bone loss [6, 7]. All known etiological factors for decreased bone mass, apart from a direct effect on bone metabolism, will indirectly affect bone via a decrease in muscle mass [7]. Apart from low BMD and low lean body mass, a higher fat mass has been reported in children with rheumatic diseases [8]. The term rheumatic cachexia refers to abnormalities in body composition with an increase in fat mass in children with rheumatic arthritis.

Effects of Growth Hormone Treatment on Body Composition in Health and Disease

In growth hormone (GH)-deficient children, GH replacement not only increases height, but also positively affects bone mass and mineral metabolism. Patients with GH deficiency exhibit abnormal body composition with low muscle mass and increased fat mass. With GH administration, body composition normalizes [9]. Protein catabolism, a common side effect in patients receiving GCs, may also be attenuated by GH administration, which has been shown to decrease amino acid catabolism and stimulate protein synthesis in both healthy volunteers and chronically ill patients [10, 11].

Effects of GH on Bone Metabolism and Bone Mass in Patients with JIA

Studies of recombinant human GH treatment in patients with JIA show an increase in height as well as a positive effect on bone metabolism and BMD [12–14]. In a 4-year study, Bechtold et al. showed that GH treatment in patients with JIA resulted in increased growth velocity, increased height and height-corrected BMD as measured by dual-energy X-ray absorptiometry (DEXA) [15]. Densitometry data obtained by DEXA are greatly influenced

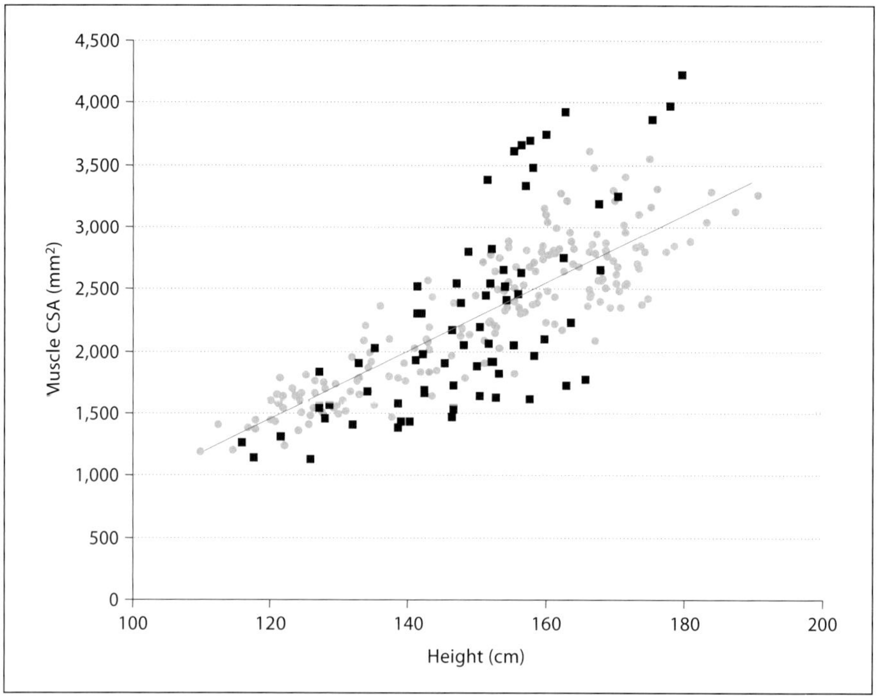

Fig. 2. Relationship between muscle mass and height during long-term treatment with growth hormone in patients with juvenile idiopathic arthritis (indicated by black squares). Gray dots represent a healthy reference population and the gray line represents the mean for boys and girls. CSA = Cross-sectional area.

by bone size; therefore, children's growth must be studied longitudinally. One possible approach is the use of volumetric BMD (vBMD), in which areal BMD (aBMD) data are derived from DEXA using the formula developed by Kröger and colleagues [16]: vBMD = aBMD [4/(π · width)].

Using this formula, Bechtold et al. found that the increase in vBMD over 4 years in patients with JIA was modest and within normal range for chronological age and bone age. However, the bone stabilization and avoidance of further bone loss noted during GH treatment could be considered beneficial effects [15].

Studies have also shown that, in response to GH treatment, patients with JIA have increased levels of alkaline phosphatase, plasma C-terminal propeptide of type I collagen and plasma insulin-like growth factor I. Serum and urinary calcium levels varied with no substantial changes noted. Markers of osteoclast activity (i.e., deoxypyridinoline) were diminished, but following GH treatment, they increased and remained within normal levels. Since there was a net increase in BMD [13–15], bone formation stimulated by GH must outweigh bone resorption.

Peripheral quantitative computed tomography allows cross-sectional imaging of the limb to permit real, volumetric, 3-dimensional assessment of the structural and geometric properties of the appendicular skeleton. Thus, it provides a more detailed insight into bone geometry. We have used it to assess longitudinal changes in trabecular bone in patients with JIA who were receiving GC treatment and noted no changes in BMD. In most patients, BMD remained within normal limits (fig. 1). Metaphyseal and diaphyseal total bone cross-sectional areas were significantly greater in the GH-treated group when compared with an age-matched control group of patients with JIA after 4 years of GH treatment ($p < 0.05$). BMC, a bone strength parameter, and the strength strain index, a combination of architectural and material components of bone stability, were significantly greater ($p < 0.05$). The increased bone size was due to periosteal bone apposition together with a greater expansion of the medullary cavity, possibly resulting in greater bone stability [17].

Effects of GH on Body Composition in JIA

Although patients with JIA experience a reduction in total BMD and bone geometry in combination with short stature, longitudinal data confirm that the main contributor to errant bone maturation in JIA is reduced muscle mass and force [18]. Thus, apart from its efficacy in disease control, GH treatment might be beneficial in these patients by positively influencing muscle development [10, 11].

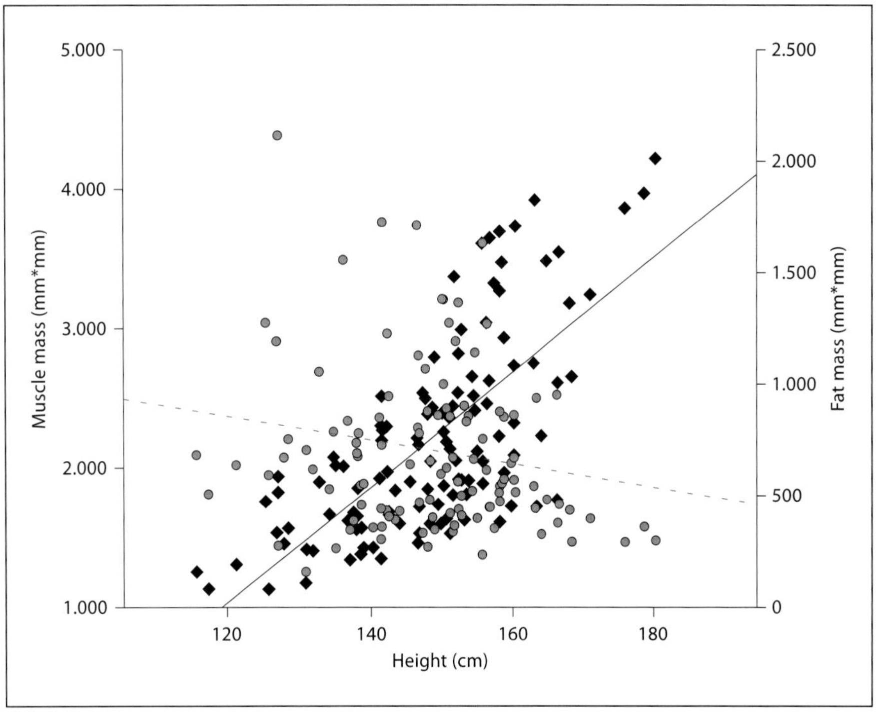

Fig. 3. Anabolic effects of growth hormone (GH) treatment: longitudinal development of muscle mass (indicated by black diamonds) and fat mass in relation to height (indicated by gray dots). With GH treatment, there is an increase in muscle mass ($R^2 = 0.505$) and a parallel decrease in fat mass ($R^2 = 0.033$).

Muscle size is negatively affected by GC therapy. Patients with JIA who received long-term treatment with GH showed a significant ($p < 0.01$) increase in muscle mass in relation to height (fig. 2). When compared with an untreated control group of JIA patients, muscle mass was 1.5 times greater in JIA patients who received GH therapy. The larger the muscle mass, the higher the total bone cross-sectional area, resulting in a higher BMC [17, 19].

Alterations in body composition have been described in patients with rheumatoid arthritis. Children with JIA, especially the more severe forms, gained less lean body mass and more fat mass and had lower BMC when compared with healthy controls [20]. Whether treatment with GH as an anabolic agent could mitigate these side effects was unclear. Touati et al. [13] demonstrated reduced fat mass and increased lean body mass during the first year of GH treatment, which was reversible after discontinuation of GH treatment. Simon et al. showed that, during 3 years of GH treatment, lean body mass steadily increased and fat mass decreased as measured by DEXA in children with JIA who required steroid treatment [19]. In a similar setting over 4 years, muscle cross-sectional area increased significantly and relative fat cross-sectional area decreased significantly ($p < 0.05$) in GH-treated patients over time (fig. 3) [17].

Conclusions

The effects of GH treatment in patients with severe forms of JIA, such as polyarticular and systemic JIA, are promising since GH treatment not only improves height velocity and final height, but also positively affects bone density, bone metabolism, bone geometry and body composition. Variables, including disease severity, GC dosage and delayed or slowed progression of puberty, influence the response to GH treatment. Long-term studies are needed to evaluate the impact of GH treatment on body composition at final height. Additionally, the long-term consequences of GH treatment on glucose metabolism in patients with JIA receiving GCs need to be evaluated. Adequate follow-up and optimal treatment of patients with JIA will require close collaboration between endocrinologists and rheumatologists.

Disclosure Statement

S.B. declares no conflict of interest. R.D.P. declares no conflict of interest. H.P.S. received grant support from Pfizer Inc. from 2000 to 2005. D.S. declares no conflict of interest.

References

1 Rauch F: Geometric strength: bone size during skeletal development. Curr Opin Endocrinol Diabetes 2006;13:10–14.
2 Rauch F: Bone growth in length and width: the yin and yang of bone stability. J Musculoskelet Neuronal Interact 2005;5:194–201.
3 Schönau E, Neu CM, Beck B, Manz F, Rauch F: Bone mineral content per muscle cross-sectional area as an index of the functional muscle-bone unit. J Bone Miner Res 2002;17:1095–1101.
4 Kontaniemi A: Growth retardation and bone loss as determinants of axial osteopenia in juvenile chronic arthritis. Scand J Rheumatol 1997;26:14–18.
5 Hendersson CJ, Specker BL, Sierra RI, Campaigne BN, Lovell DJ: Total body bone mineral content in non-corticosteroid-treated postpubertal females with juvenile rheumatoid arthritis. Arthritis Rheum 2000;43:531–540.
6 Bechtold S, Ripperger P, Dalla Pozza R, Schmidt H, Häfner R, Schwarz HP: Musculoskeletal and functional muscle-bone analysis in children with rheumatic disease using peripheral quantitative computed tomography. Osteoporos Int 2005;16:757–763.
7 Roth J, Palm C, Scheunemann I, Ranke MB, Schweizer R, Dannecker GE: Musculoskeletal abnormalities of the forearm in patients with juvenile idiopathic arthritis relate mainly to bone geometry. Arthritis Rheum 2004;50:1277–1285.
8 Mul D, van Suijlekom-Smit LW, ten Cate R, Bekkering WP, de Muinck Keizer-Schrama SM: Bone mineral density and body composition and influencing factors in children with rheumatic diseases treated with corticosteroids. J Pediatr Endocrinol Metab 2002;15:187–192.
9 Högler W, Briody J, Moore B, Lu PW, Cowell CT: Effect of growth hormone therapy and puberty on bone and body composition in children with idiopathic short stature and growth hormone deficiency. Bone 2005;37:642–650.
10 Berneis K, Ninnis R, Girard J, Frey B, Keller U: Effects of insulin like growth factor I combined with growth hormone on glucocorticoid-induced whole body protein catabolism in man. J Clin Endocrinol Metab 1997;82:2528–2534.
11 Horber FF, Haymond MW: Human growth hormone prevents the protein catabolic side effects of prednisone in humans. J Clin Invest 1990;86:265–272.
12 Bechtold S, Ripperger P, Mühlbayer, Truckenbrodt H, Häfner R, Butenandt O, Schwarz HP: GH therapy in juvenile chronic arthritis: results of a two year controlled study on growth and bone. J Clin Endocrinol Metab 2001;86:5737–5744.
13 Touati G, Ruiz JC, Porquet D, Kindermans C, Prieur AM, Czernichow P: Effects on bone metabolism of one year recombinant human growth hormone administration to children with juvenile chronic arthritis undergoing chronic steroid therapy. J Rheumatol 2000;27:1287–1293.
14 Rooney M, Davies UM, Reeve J, Preece M, Ansell BM, Woo PM: Bone mineral content and bone mineral metabolism: changes after growth hormone treatment in juvenile chronic arthritis. J Rheumatol 2000;27:1073–1081.
15 Bechtold S, Ripperger P, Bonfig W, Schmidt H, Bitterling H, Häfner R, Schwarz HP: Bone mass development and bone metabolism in juvenile idiopathic arthritis: treatment with growth hormone for 4 years. J Rheumatol 2004;31:1407–1412.
16 Kröger H, Vainio P, Nieminen J, Kontaniemi A: Comparison of different models for interpreting bone mineral density measurements using DXA and MRI technology. Bone 1995;17:157–159.
17 Bechtold S, Ripperger P, Bonfig W, Dalla Pozza R, Haefner R, Schwarz HP: Growth hormone changes bone geometry and body composition in patients with juvenile idiopathic arthritis requiring glucocorticoid treatment: a controlled study using peripheral quantitative computed tomography. J Clin Endocrinol Metab 2005;90:3168–3173.
18 Roth J, Linge M, Tzaribachev N, Schweizer R, Kuemmerle-Deschner J: Musculoskeletal abnormalities in juvenile idiopathic arthritis – a 4-year longitudinal study. Rheumatology 2007;46:1180–1184.
19 Simon D, Lucidarme N, Prieur AM, Ruiz JC, Czernichow P: Effects on growth and body composition of growth hormone treatment in children with juvenile idiopathic arthritis requiring steroid therapy. J Rheumatol 2003;30:2492–2499.
20 Lien G, Selvaag AM, Flatø B, Haugen M, Vinje O, Sørskaar D, Dale K, Egeland T, Førre Ø: A two-year prospective controlled study of bone mass and bone turnover in children with early juvenile idiopathic arthritis. Arthritis Rheumatol 2005;52:833–840.

HORMONE RESEARCH

Horm Res 2009;72(suppl 1):65–68
DOI: 10.1159/000229767

Published online: November 27, 2009

Safety of Growth Hormone Treatment in Children with Juvenile Idiopathic Arthritis

Dominique Simon

Department of Endocrinology and Diabetology, Hôpital Robert Debré, Paris, France

Key Words
Juvenile idiopathic arthritis · Growth hormone · Glucocorticoids · Glucose tolerance

Abstract
Background: Available data on growth hormone (GH) therapy in glucocorticoid-treated children with juvenile idiopathic arthritis (JIA) suggest a satisfactory safety profile. There have been few reports of adverse effects on the course of the joint disease (e.g., inflammatory flare-ups or osteo-articular complications). Despite strong concern that combined glucocorticoid and GH therapy might impair glucose tolerance, this has been uncommon in clinical trials. This article briefly reviews the published data and offers recommendations for monitoring patients with JIA who are receiving GH replacement therapy. ***Conclusions:*** The safety of GH therapy in children receiving glucocorticoid therapy for JIA seems satisfactory with few serious adverse events reported to date; however, given the small number of treated patients and the short periods of follow-up in each individual patient, the decision to initiate GH therapy in patients receiving glucocorticoids should be made cautiously.

Introduction

Safety is of crucial concern when using growth hormone (GH) in new indications, most notably in children with chronic diseases. This article reviews key published data on the safety of GH therapy in glucocorticoid-treated children with juvenile idiopathic arthritis (JIA). The potential effects of GH therapy on the natural history of JIA and the risk of GH-induced diabetes in this high-risk population will be emphasized.

Influence of GH Therapy on the Course of JIA

Systemic Inflammation

Although GH interacts with the immune system [1–3], recent analysis of a large database of GH-treated patients indicates no immunological anomalies attributable to GH treatment [4]. However, it was important during clinical trials to determine if GH therapy had any impact on the progression of JIA. Clinical variables (e.g., the number of tender and swollen joints, physical assessment by the physician and family and number of flare-ups), laboratory tests (e.g., erythrocyte sedimentation rate, C-reactive protein, blood cell and platelet counts and fibrin level) and therapeutic variables (e.g., changes over time in the dosages of glucocorticoids and other antirheumatic medications) are used to assess disease activity. In the

KARGER

Fax +41 61 306 12 34
E-Mail karger@karger.ch
www.karger.com

0301–0163/09/0727–0065$26.00/0

Accessible online at:
www.karger.com/hre

Dr. Dominique Simon
Department of Endocrinology and Diabetology, Hôpital Robert Debré
48, boulevard Sérurier, FR–75019 Paris (France)
Tel. +33 1 40 03 3634, Fax +33 1 40 03 2429
E-Mail dominique.simon@rdb.aphp.fr

Table 1. Effects of growth hormone treatment on glucose and plasma insulin levels in patients (n = 13) receiving glucocorticoid therapy for juvenile idiopathic arthritis

OGTT	Baseline	Year 1	Year 2	Year 3
Serum glucose, mmol/l				
Time 0	3.9 (3.1, 4.9)	4.1 (3.4, 5.1)	4.6 (3.6, 5.5)	4.4 (3.2, 5.2)
Time 120 min	5.8 (4.8, 6.7)	6.8 (3.7, 9.2)	$7.1^{*,\dagger}$ (4.5, 9.9)	7.0* (4.9, 8.8)
Plasma insulin, mU/l				
Time 0	10 (3, 29)	14 (3, 37)	10.6 (3, 180)	11.1 (4, 29)
Time 120 min	55 (15, 157)	107 (4, 721)	112 (13, 442)	91 (9, 322)
Hemoglobin A_{1c}, %	5.5 (5, 6.6)	5.8 (5.3, 6.0)	5.6 (4.9, 6.1)	5.8 (4.7, 6.4)

Reprinted from Simon et al. [9] with permission from The Journal of Rheumatology. OGTT = Oral glucose tolerance test. Values are expressed as medians (range).

* $p < 0.05$ versus baseline values; † $p < 0.05$ versus values in the previous year (nonparametric Wilcoxon signed rank test).

randomized controlled trials published to date, patients were followed for up to 7 years, and no substantial differences were found in disease activity variables between GH-treated patients and control subjects [5–11]. Although relapses were observed during GH therapy, no demonstrable link was made to GH. One patient who experienced a flare-up of JIA during GH therapy discontinued GH treatment at the family's request.

Osteoarticular Complications

Focal growth disorders may occur near affected joints in children with JIA. Thus, epiphyseal hypertrophy predominating at the medial femoral condyle may induce *genu valgum*, or 'knock-knees'. Growth plate stimulation at the knee may lead to limb length inequality. Early growth plate closure at the hindfoot or hand may result in shortening of the foot or metacarpals. Furthermore, the systemic effects of chronic inflammation and glucocorticoid therapy may adversely affect bone mineralization, and as a result, vertebral fractures may occur during the active phase of the disease. All of these osteoarticular complications can substantially impair function and ultimately outcome in patients with JIA.

GH stimulates linear bone growth. Bone mineralization is enhanced via a biphasic effect on bone remodeling that consists of increased bone resorption followed by increased bone formation. The net result is an increase in bone mass. In clinical trials, clinical variables and imaging studies were used to determine whether GH therapy influenced bone deformities and vertebral fractures via stimulation of linear bone growth and bone mineralization, respectively.

GH therapy was not associated with worsening of preexisting bone deformities. In a randomized controlled trial of 31 patients, lumbar lordosis and moderate scoliosis developed in similar numbers of treated and untreated patients during follow-up [11]. In our randomized study of 30 patients, neither the treated nor the untreated patients had clinical or radiological evidence of changes in vertebral alignment during the 3-year follow-up [10]. At baseline, three treated and two untreated patients each had one vertebral fracture, and two treated patients each experienced one vertebral fracture during the study period [10]. Other osteoarticular complications reported during GH therapy included Legg-Calvé-Perthes disease and osteochondritis. A single patient with JIA who experienced a favorable outcome of hip osteochondritis during GH therapy has been reported [8]. No other cases of Legg-Calvé-Perthes disease have been described to date in patients with JIA treated with GH.

Available data indicate that GH therapy probably has no substantial effect on the evolution of JIA. Nevertheless, the endocrinologist and the physician managing the joint disease must work closely together during follow-up. The endocrinologist should be apprised of the clinical and radiological parameters used to monitor joint status, relevant laboratory tests for inflammation and any changes in treatment. This information is necessary for assessing the quality of the treatment response and detecting adverse reactions that could be attributed to GH administration.

Fig. 1. Changes in oral glucose tolerance in a boy who developed diabetes mellitus during a relapse of JIA. Oral glucose tolerance was normal before starting GH treatment (65 µg/kg/day). After 2 years of GH treatment, the patient experienced a severe relapse of JIA that required initiation of high-dose prednisone therapy (0.95 mg/kg/day). The patient subsequently developed asymptomatic diabetes. GH dosages were then decreased by 40%, and 3 months later, oral glucose tolerance parameters normalized. Note that fasting glycemia remained normal.

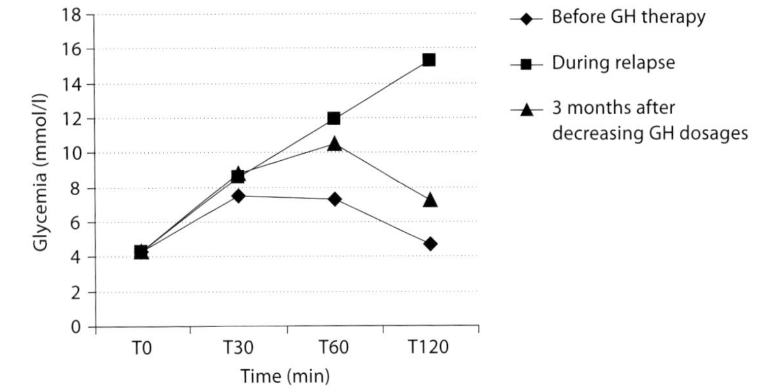

Effect of GH Therapy on Glucose Tolerance

Children with JIA are at risk for impaired glucose homeostasis, as both chronic inflammation and glucocorticoid treatment substantially decrease sensitivity to insulin [12–14]. GH also decreases sensitivity to insulin [15, 16]. However, among patients given supraphysiological doses of GH for such conditions as intrauterine growth retardation or Turner syndrome, none experienced severe disturbances in glucose homeostasis [17, 18]. In children receiving glucocorticoid therapy for JIA, glucose tolerance is typically monitored using blood glucose, fasting insulin and glycated hemoglobin assays at 6- to 12-month intervals. Optimal monitoring involves oral glucose tolerance tests (OGTT) at baseline and then once yearly during treatment. In GH-treated patients, increased insulin resistance manifested as high fasting and poststimulation insulin levels, with or without changes in fasting blood glucose or glycated hemoglobin levels, was a consistent finding [8, 19]. All these abnormalities resolved after GH discontinuation. In long-term studies, a few patients experienced transient glucose intolerance or asymptomatic diabetes [9, 10] diagnosed by OGTT (table 1). In patients with glucose tolerance impairment, this abnormality usually occurred during puberty or during JIA relapses requiring substantial glucocorticoid dose increases. Glucose tolerance normalized when the dosage of glucocorticoid and/or GH was diminished. No patient required insulin therapy. These data indicate that patients on long-term glucocorticoid therapy should receive close monitoring with OGTT and glycated hemoglobin assays at baseline, then once yearly during GH therapy. If diabetes develops, the GH dose should be decreased; persistent diabetes may necessitate discontinuation of GH therapy. Figure 1 shows changes in OGTT in a boy who developed diabetes mellitus during a relapse of JIA. With a 40% reduction in GH dosage, results of his OGTT normalized.

When a severe flare-up of JIA occurs, temporary discontinuation of GH therapy may decrease the risk of glucose homeostasis impairment. During periods of severe inflammation, GH has little effect on growth; therefore, stopping GH therapy during severe flare-ups should not negate any gains in linear growth.

Monitoring Other Aspects of GH Therapy in Children with JIA

Long-term glucocorticoid therapy may increase the risk of water and sodium retention during GH therapy. No cases of intracranial hypertension have been reported in GH-treated children with JIA. Nevertheless, it is better to start GH therapy at a low dosage followed by a slow increase, especially in patients taking large amounts of glucocorticoids.

When administering supraphysiological dosages of GH, clinicians should monitor serum IGF-I levels since patients with JIA also take multiple immunosuppressant medications that can increase tumor risk. Serum IGF-I levels tend to be lower in patients with JIA [20, 21] because inflammation induces resistance to GH [22–24]. With GH therapy, serum IGF-I levels increase substantially, but remain correlated with disease activity [11] and within the therapeutic range currently recommended for patients on GH therapy.

Conclusions

The safety profile of GH seems satisfactory in children receiving glucocorticoid therapy for JIA. Few serious adverse effects have been reported to date; however, the number of treated patients is small and the length of follow-up is short. Close monitoring of endocrine function in conjunction with managing the joint disease during and after GH therapy is necessary to evaluate any possible effects of GH treatment on the natural history of JIA. Metabolic complications (e.g., glucose intolerance and diabetes) are usually asymptomatic and should therefore be investigated routinely. The potential long-term effects of GH-induced hyperinsulinism should be assessed by metabolic tests shortly after treatment discontinuation.

Disclosure Statement

The author has received honoraria from Pfizer.

References

1 Savino W, Postel-Vinay MC, Smaniotto S, Dardenne M: The thymus gland: a target organ for growth hormone. Scand J Immunol 2002;55:442–452.
2 Manfredi R, Tumietto F, Azzaroli L, Zucchini A, Chiodo F, Manfredi G: Growth hormone (GH) and the immune system: impaired phagocytic function in children with idiopathic GH deficiency is corrected by treatment with biosynthetic GH. J Pediatr Endocrinol 1994;7:245–251.
3 Bozzola M, De Benedetti F, De Amici M, Jouret B, Travaglino P, Pagani S, Conte F, Tauber M: Stimulating effect of growth hormone on cytokine release in children. Eur J Endocrinol 2003;149:397–401.
4 Wilson P. Adverse events reported in KIGS; in Ranke MB, Price DA, Reiter EO (eds): Growth Hormone Therapy in Pediatrics – 20 Years of KIGS. Basel, Karger, 2007, pp 432–441.
5 Svantesson H: Treatment of growth failure with human growth hormone in patients with juvenile chronic arthritis. A pilot study. Clin Exp Rheumatol 1991;9(suppl 6):47–50.
6 Davies UM, Rooney M, Preece MA, Ansell BM, Woo P: Treatment of growth retardation in juvenile chronic arthritis with recombinant human growth hormone. J Rheumatol 1994;21:153–158.
7 Bechtold S, Ripperger P, Häfner R, Said E, Schwarz HP: Growth hormone improves height in patients with juvenile idiopathic arthritis: 4-year data of a controlled study. J Pediatr 2003;143:512–519.
8 Touati G, Prieur AM, Ruiz JC, Noel M, Czernichow P: Beneficial effects of one-year growth hormone administration to children with juvenile chronic arthritis on chronic steroid therapy. I. Effects on growth velocity and body composition. J Clin Endocrinol Metab 1998;83:403–409.
9 Simon D, Lucidarme N, Prieur AM, Ruiz JC, Czernichow P: Effects on growth and body composition of growth hormone treatment in children with juvenile idiopathic arthritis requiring steroid therapy. J Rheumatol 2003; 30:2492–2499.
10 Simon D, Prieur AM, Quartier P, Charles Ruiz J, Czernichow P: Early recombinant human growth hormone treatment in glucocorticoid-treated children with juvenile idiopathic arthritis: a 3-year randomized study. J Clin Endocrinol Metab 2007;92: 2567–2573.
11 Bechtold S, Ripperger P, Dalla Pozza R, Bonfig W, Häfner R, Michels H, Schwarz HP: Growth hormone increases final height in patients with juvenile idiopathic arthritis: data from a randomized controlled study. J Clin Endocrinol Metab 2007;92:3013–3018.
12 Tsigos C, Papanicolaou DA, Defensor R, Mitsiadis CS, Kyrou I, Chrousos GP: Dose effects of recombinant human interleukin-6 on pituitary hormone secretion and energy expenditure. Neuroendocrinology 1997;66: 54–62.
13 Pittas AG, Joseph NA, Greenberg AS: Adipocytokines and insulin resistance. J Clin Endocrinol Metab 2004;89:447–452.
14 Rizza RA, Mandarino LJ, Gerich JE: Cortisol-induced insulin resistance in man: impaired suppression of glucose production and stimulation of glucose utilization due to a postreceptor detect of insulin action. J Clin Endocrinol Metab 1982;54:131–138.
15 Bratusch-Marrain PR, Smith D, DeFronzo RA: The effect of growth hormone on glucose metabolism and insulin secretion in man. J Clin Endocrinol Metab 1982;55:973–982.
16 Horber FF, Marsh HM, Haymond MW: Differential effects of prednisone and growth hormone on fuel metabolism and insulin antagonism in humans. Diabetes 1991;40:141–149.
17 Sas T, de Muinck Keizer-Schrama S, Aanstoot HJ, Stijnen T, Drop S: Carbohydrate metabolism during growth hormone treatment and after discontinuation of growth hormone treatment in girls with Turner syndrome treated with once or twice daily growth hormone injections. Clin Endocrinol (Oxford) 2000;52:741–747.
18 Sas T, Mulder P, Aanstoot HJ, Houdijk M, Jansen M, Reeser M, Hokken-Koelega A: Carbohydrate metabolism during long-term growth hormone treatment in children with short stature born small for gestational age. Clin Endocrinol (Oxford) 2001;54:243–251.
19 Allen DB, Julius JR, Breen TJ, Attie KM: Treatment of glucocorticoid-induced growth suppression with growth hormone. National Cooperative Growth Study. J Clin Endocrinol Metab 1998;83:2824–2829.
20 Allen RC, Jimenez M, Cowell CT: Insulin-like growth factor and growth hormone secretion in juvenile chronic arthritis. Ann Rheum Dis 1991;50:602–606.
21 Bennett AE, Silverman ED, Miller JJ 3rd, Hintz RL: Insulin-like growth factors I and II in children with systemic onset juvenile arthritis. J Rheumatol 1988;15:655–658.
22 Thissen JP, Verniers J: Inhibition by interleukin-1 beta and tumor necrosis factor-alpha of the insulin-like growth factor I messenger ribonucleic acid response to growth hormone in rat hepatocyte primary culture. Endocrinology 1997;138:1078–1084.
23 Bergad PL, Schwarzenberg SJ, Humbert JT, Morrison M, Amarasinghe S, Towle HC, Berry SA: Inhibition of growth hormone action in models of inflammation. Am J Physiol Cell Physiol 2000;279:C1906–C1917.
24 Yumet G, Shumate ML, Bryant P, Lin CM, Lang CH, Cooney RN: Tumor necrosis factor mediates hepatic growth hormone resistance during sepsis. Am J Physiol Endocrinol Metab 2002;283:E472–E481.

HORMONE
RESEARCH

Author Index Vol. 72, Suppl. 1, 2009

KARGER

Fax +41 61 306 12 34
E-Mail karger@karger.ch
www.karger.com

Accessible online at:
www.karger.com/hre

HORMONE
RESEARCH

Subject Index Vol. 72, Suppl. 1, 2009

KARGER

Fax +41 61 306 12 34
E-Mail karger@karger.ch
www.karger.com

Accessible online at:
www.karger.com/hre

A comprehensive review on psychiatric and gynecologic aspects

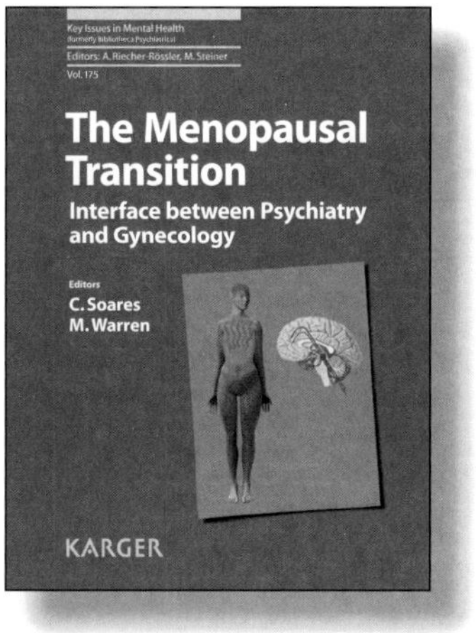

The Menopausal Transition

Interface between Gynecology and Psychiatry

Editors
Claudio Soares
Michelle Warren

Psychiatry, Gynecology, Neuroendocrinology, Pharmacology, Psychology

The interplay of hormones, health and behavior across the female life cycle, especially during the menopausal transition, poses a special challenge to health care professionals.
Written by experts, this book brings together the knowledge gained on the menopausal transition from clinical experience and medical research. Topics like 'what to expect' from the menopausal transition, sexuality, sociocultural changes, impact of life stressors, and emergence of depression are discussed. The physiology of thermoregulation and the occurrence of hot flashes are reviewed to promote a better understanding of vasomotor complaints. Another chapter offers an update on hormonal and nonhormonal treatment strategies by presenting an overview of the management of mood and anxiety during the menopausal transition. The emergence of psychotic symptoms associated with peri- and postmenopausal changes in sex hormone levels is also addressed. Lastly, the book includes an excellent review on the pros and cons of hormonal therapy in the post-Women's Health Initiative era.
This book is essential for gynecologists, psychiatrists, endocrinologists, epidemiologists involved in the clinical care of mature women as well as researchers and students interested in obtaining an up-to-date overview of this topic.

KI 09432

Contents

www.karger.com/kismh

Key Issues in Mental Health, Vol. 175
Series Editor: Riecher-Rössler, A. (Basel); Steiner, M. (Hamilton, Ont.)
ISSN 1662–4874 / e-ISSN 1662–4882

The Menopausal Transition
Interface between Gynecoloy and Psychiatry
Editors: Soares, C. (Hamilton, Ont.); Warren, M. (New York, N.Y.)
VIII + 150 p., 9 fig., 4 in color, 5 tab., hard cover, 2009
CHF 64.– / EUR 46.– / USD 64.00
Prices subject to change
EUR price for Germany, USD price for USA only
ISBN 978–3–8055–9101–0
e-ISBN 978–3–8055–9102–7

KARGER

Order Form

Please send: ______ copy/ies

Postage and handling free with prepayment

Payment:
Please charge to my credit card
☐ American Express ☐ Diners ☐ Eurocard
☐ MasterCard ☐ Visa

Card No.: ____________________

Exp. date: ____________________

CVV/CVC ____________________
(3 digits in the signature field on the back of Visa and MasterCard)

☐ Check enclosed ☐ Please bill me

Orders may be placed with any bookshop, subscription agency, directly with the publisher or through a Karger distributor.

Fax: +41 61 306 12 34

S. Karger AG, P.O. Box, CH–4009 Basel (Switzerland)
E-Mail orders@karger.ch, **www.karger.com**

Name/Address: ____________________

Date: ____________________

Signature: ____________________